SURVIVING THE STORM WITHIN

Life with Lyme Disease

Kristin Parthemos

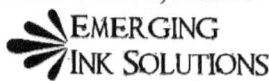

This book is dedicated to my dear friend, Whitney Paige Shelton, who not only taught me the true meaning of friendship but is one of the best people I have ever been blessed to know.

A gentle soul, she was diagnosed at the age of thirty-nine with Hereditary Sensory and Autonomic Neuropathy (HSAN) Type 1E, a slowly progressive neurological disorder.

So, to Whitney—Thank you for the laughter, the secrets we shared, and all that makes you unique and wonderful.

Table of Contents

Chronic illness affects millions of people worldwide. It is one of the greatest challenges many face today.

Those suffering from chronic illness often feel completely abandoned. It is my wish that this book eases their despair and helps them feel less alone.

Preface

A SUNNY DAY IS NEVER promised.

Weather can be unpredictable, replacing the sun with heavy rain and robust winds. Dark, gloomy skies abound. The air turns frigid, the wind whips in anger, and thunder booms, rattling the Earth. There is no escaping the storm as rain hammers at your window and flashes of lightning seep through the curtains. The wind grows stronger and the movements of the earth more violent, flooding your senses with the overpowering howl of gusts.

Blustery weather forces its way inside, tearing off the roof and disintegrating the walls. Outside with no protection, the rain consumes you, obscuring your vision. The sudden decrease in air pressure causes unthinkable pain, and you worry you may go deaf. Dropping to your knees and covering your ears, you scream out in pain. No one hears you. Soaked to the bone, you begin to shiver and shake. Attempting to crawl to safety, your breathing becomes slow and shallow. Your thoughts are foggy and your skin turns blue. Tormented, you wonder if this pain, this terror, will ever end. Will the skies calm again?

This is life with chronic illness. Without warning, new symptoms come barreling through your body like a tornado, whipping across your beautiful life to leave nothing but debris and damage in their wake. Sure, you can rebuild, and you always try. But you're tired. There's no one to warn you when the storm is coming, and there's no one to help you navigate it or rebuild once it passes.

You don't know how long it will last, how bad it will be, or if you'll be able to continue to rebuild each time. There is only one choice when chronic illness rears its ugly head—hunker down and weather the storm. Do your best to make it through the worst of times. When the storm lets up, even for just a little while, look for the sun. See its powerful rays peering through the clouds. Embrace its brilliance. Stand outside and feel the returning warmth on your skin. Enjoy this gift of beauty and wonder you've been given.

Put your hand on your chest, feel the beating of your heart, and know you're alive. Remember, you are a warrior. You can handle anything, and you will. But weathering storms of chronic illness is difficult and might seem pointless. How do we go about remaining strong during the worst of winds? How do we survive in a world where chronic illness is so misunderstood?

Education, support, persistence, and self-love are key to survival. Find one person who can guide or support you on your journey. This could be a loved one, a friend, a counselor, a doctor, or a health coach. Stay educated, ask questions, never give up, and locate a doctor who fights for you and possesses empathy and understanding of your plight. None of these things come easily, but all are part of my journey that unfolds within the pages of this book.

My expedition involves a dark road paved with one of the most deeply misunderstood chronic illnesses—Lyme disease. Lyme disease and the co-infections that often come along with the bite of a tick, flea, fly, mite, or mosquito continue to be illnesses of silent suffering. [1] Many of us with Lyme disease find ourselves secluded and in agony—alone and scared—fearful that our lives will end, or that we will never get back to the person we once were.

Once you're led down this dark and lonely road, you are forever altered and molded into a new version of yourself. Tattered and worn from multiple storms, you become stronger, wiser, and empathetic of the struggles of others. These changes do not indicate the previous version of you has disappeared, only that you have emerged as a new you. A different you. A version that is just as important as the last.

---

[1] "At least nine species of ticks, six species of mosquitos, 13 species of mites, 15 species of flies, two species of fleas, and numerous wild and domestic animals (including rabbits, rodents, and birds) have been found to carry the spirochete that causes Lyme disease" (Virginia Lyme, "How Many Species of Ticks Carry the Lyme disease Spirochetes?" Accessed September 23, 2022, https://sites.google.com/site/virginialyme/faq.)

However, according to the CDC, "There is no credible evidence that Lyme disease bacteria can be transmitted through air, food, water, or from the bites of mosquitoes, flies, fleas, or lice," (Center for Disease Control and Prevention, "Transmission," January 20, 2023, https://rb.gy/o1vpt.)

Within this book, I'll discuss how I've pushed myself to live my life and not let chronic illness consume me. At times, it is difficult, but the stories contained herein are the moments that shaped me, transformed me, and guided me to become the person I am today. I will remind you now and many more times: you are not your disease. You are *you*.

We are all individuals worthy of love. Being you is a special gift that only you bring to the world, and that alone is enough to never give up. Live your life to the fullest and find beauty in everything you can.

While I certainly do not have all the answers, what I can do is share my story with the hope that it will bring you comfort. Every person has their own tale to tell and knowledge to share. We can learn from each other, support each other, and educate others so they may not share our plight. To do better, we must know better—spreading awareness and sharing our experiences are key.

For most of us, Lyme disease begins with a host of unexplained symptoms. Without ever seeing a tick attached or a bull's-eye rash and without accurate testing, we are left in the dark searching for answers.

This book is overflowing with raw emotion and recollections of the torment that I—and my loved ones—suffered because of Lyme disease. Take my hand as I guide you through that torment, stepping into the world of suffering and sorrow that so many face every day. A world where we learn as we go, educate to survive, persist and insist, and prosper and grow. Stuck in a medical system that would rather leave us for dead, we band together to strive for change. Although we follow our own paths and experience our own pain and suffering, we share similar stories of poor treatment and being made to feel as if we're wrong, or worse—that we're crazy.

I hope my story adds another voice to the collective pursuit for change and brings comfort, knowledge, and understanding to readers.

While it may seem like you are alone, that is far from the truth. Share a brief synopsis of your story at mylymevoice@gmail.com and let it be heard.

1

And So, It Begins

PUSHING THE GAS PEDAL TOWARD the floor, I accelerated faster and faster... 55... 65... 85... 90. Closing my eyes tightly, I imagined crashing into a large building, maybe my doctor's office. Yes, my doctor's office! I wanted it to happen.

As I gripped the steering wheel and clenched my teeth, I felt rage swell inside me. It was so powerful and consuming that I could've screamed! I opened my eyes as the car accelerated faster and faster... 100... 115... speeding by several vehicles. The pain, fatigue, and exhaustion were too much to bear, and I wanted it all to end.

Rolling down the windows and feeling the wind flow through my hair felt like my last moments. This was it, and I was at peace with that. As I crossed over a bridge and looked down at the traffic below me, I realized it was in fact the road that led to my doctor's office. A sinister snicker escaped from my lips.

I looked back at the speedometer... 125. Then, a sudden thought. *What am I doing? Snap out of it!* Fear and regret unexpectedly pierced my mind. I pressed the brake pedal and reduced my speed just as I approached traffic at a stop light. My car came to a screeching halt, forcing me to stare at the brake lights in front of me.

The red lights glared at me as if they represented the evil that had just occurred. I couldn't take my eyes off them. I was frozen. The traffic light turned green, and cars moved forward—but I didn't move. Vehicles began passing me. Finally, I shook off the trance and pulled my car off to the side of the road. My hands trembled on the steering wheel as I took a deep breath to calm myself. It was a conscious effort to loosen my grip. *What is going on? This isn't me.*

I threw open the door and stepped out onto the pavement. As I leaned against the side of my car and clutched my chest, sobs erupted from my body.

I ran my fingers through my hair and glowered at the ground. My legs were unsteady, my body weak. When I looked up to take another deep breath, something caught my eye—a lovely bird soaring above me.

I wanted to be that bird so badly. To soar high, free, and peaceful among the white cottony clouds and the bright blue sky. I prayed that better days would come and that I would make it through this.

2

Infiltrate Your Mind

NEVER IN MY LIFE HAD I driven a car that fast. I understand now that Lyme disease will infiltrate your mind and make you do things you never thought you would. It is an enemy that advances into every crevice of your body, attacking it with corkscrew bacteria of destruction until it begins to run the show.

I fully admit that before my life took this unexpected turn, I didn't possess a deep understanding of medicine or the health challenges that people often face in this world. For the most part, as a young female, I enjoyed a life of health and energy.

Sure, I experienced devastating events in life, such as the passing of family members, an abusive and unhealthy relationship, and a family member's drug addiction, but my mind and body had never failed me quite like they did with Lyme disease.

One of my lowest moments prior to then had been the experience of poverty. Out of money and unable to buy groceries, I had shared a piece of bologna with my dog as I cried on my kitchen floor. No longer able to pay rent, I wondered where my dog and I would end up.

Around the same time in my life, I had witnessed a family member's soul suffer from drug abuse as their eyes grew cold and absent. The person I knew and loved was gone and addiction had taken hold. This addiction had wrapped itself tightly around the core of their being, snuffing out any trace of what made them who they were.

Now, it was my turn.

Lyme disease began invading my mind and soul, slowly increasing its grip to suffocate my very essence. Looking into my eyes, all you could see was pain and the absence of joy. The absence of presence. The existence of chronic and persistent illness— Lyme disease.

Before chronic illness, a visit to my primary care doctor involved common issues such as a sore throat or an ear infection. The doctor would prescribe medication and I would take it no questions asked. I trusted my doctor. I believed that if there were ever anything genuinely wrong with me, my doctor was educated and would inform me of such.

I was naïve.

I soon learned how vital it is to be an informed patient and take charge of your health. You must be your own advocate and understand your body. Knowledge is power. The more you understand about yourself and the chronic illness you have been given, the more easily you will be able to navigate the complex and vast world of medicine.

3

In Sickness and in Health

WHEN YOU RECITE "IN SICKNESS and in health" at your wedding, you don't expect to be faced with the former right away. The first precious years of marriage are a time for young love to blossom, not for it to be continuously tested. The expectation, rather, is for every day to be filled with happy moments and the joy of each other's company. I wish I could say my marriage had a long honeymoon phase, but it was cruelly interrupted by a dark force I never could have anticipated.

Slowly, the magic of the wedding and the vision of a beautiful bride were replaced with illness and despair. A groom now sat by his beloved in the hospital, a wedding dress replaced by a hospital gown. There were no discussions about paint colors, home projects, traveling, or starting a family. Instead, days were filled with conversations about doctors, symptoms, and medications.

I was truly happy to be married to John, so this was not how I envisioned we would spend our days together. As I lay in a hospital bed, I looked over at the amazing man I was lucky to call my husband. We had fallen in love quickly and had a connection neither of us had anticipated.

When I met John, I was enjoying the single life after having left a long-term toxic relationship a year prior. It was my time to be young and free and to play the field. My pseudo-grandma, Patty, who was a colleague at the law firm I worked at, told me, "There are plenty of fish in the sea, and it's time to go fishing!" She had not been a fan of my ex-boyfriend and wanted me to go out in the world and enjoy myself.

I finally heeded her advice and began dating for the first time in years. I wasn't looking for a serious relationship and wanted to see what was out there. At the time, my best friend and soul sister, Liz, was also single. Despite our age difference of nearly five years, we were inseparable.

I met her when my family moved from Pennsylvania to Virginia. Liz had just turned four when I moved in across the street. She was the first kid to ring my doorbell and ask if I could come outside to play. From then on, we were practically inseparable. We shared many dinners at each other's homes and had frequent sleepovers. Liz was the most adorable and sweetest child you could ever meet. Her personality was a beautiful mixture of curiosity and softness. She was short and petite, like me, with straight dirty-blond hair that fell at her shoulders. She was always looking for acceptance and love.

When I became single, Liz met a guy named Luca and was *obsessed* with him. One night, she begged me to go with her to a party where she knew he'd be.

"Come on, Kristin. It will be fun! There is going to be a party at this guy John's house, and Luca will be there. I really want you to come with me."

"I don't know, Liz. I have a ton of schoolwork."

I was working full-time as a paralegal and going to college at night. It was a Friday night, but I felt the pressure to finish my schoolwork so I could relax for the rest of the weekend.

"Please! Maybe we can go for just a little while?"

Liz looked at me with those pouty eyes of hers and an adorable frown. She always had this way of making me do whatever she wanted. I was a sucker for her. As I said before, she was more than a best friend to me; she was a sister who annoyed the heck out of me. I absolutely adored her.

"Okay, let's go," I said reluctantly.

"Yay!"

"I'm not staying long though!" I added.

Liz nodded with a smile. "Okay, sure, that's fine."

"Let me just throw on something a little nicer and I'll be ready."

On our way to the party, Liz received a phone call. It was Luca. It sounded like plans had changed. "The party is canceled," she said once off the phone.

"What? Why?" I asked.

"I don't know, but we are going to meet them at the 7-Eleven."

"7-Eleven? What are we going to do there?"

"I don't know. We'll just meet up with them and see what their plans are now."

"Whose house did you say this was?" Liz was always getting me into these situations. She was such a carefree person.

"It's John's house. He has a townhouse and that's where the party was supposed to be, but it got canceled. Have you been listening?" Liz asked as she smoothed out her dress and lightly combed her fingers through her hair.

"You really like this guy, don't you? Quit worrying, you look great, Liz."

We pulled into the 7-Eleven, and John and Luca greeted us at the driver's-side window. I recognized Luca right away and realized I already knew him. We had met several times before, knew some of the same people, and were around the same age. When you live in a smaller town, usually everybody is connected in some fashion. I remembered him as a decent and friendly person. He was a short Italian guy with dark hair and a small build.

I flashed a grin his way. "Hey, Luca!"

"What's up, Kristin?" Luca replied with a smile. "This is John."

I glanced over at John. He had messy, sandy blond hair and blue eyes. He boasted strong, broad shoulders and a curious smile. Although he was of average height, he was a bit taller than Luca.

"Hey John, nice to meet you," I greeted.

"Nice to meet you too."

"So, what are you all up to now that the party is canceled?" I inquired.

"I don't know. Nothing I guess. Would you want to drive over to the house to hang out? We can show you where it is," Luca offered.

I glanced at Liz. "Sure, that sounds good."

"Hop in and we'll give you a ride," said Liz. Leave it to Liz to invite people into my car.

Luca and John slid into the backseat, and we drove over to John's house. It was only three blocks away and right in town. I was taken aback by how close it was. We could have walked.

When we arrived at John's place, we hung out in the kitchen and talked and laughed. We had a surprisingly great time. I never expected to enjoy myself so much, especially since I hadn't wanted to come in the first place. Luca and John were hilarious, and the conversation easily flowed. We discovered we all had a lot in common. Liz and I didn't stay more than an hour or two, and when we left, we couldn't stop talking about it.

Liz and I returned to John's a few more times to hang out and party. She spoke about Luca nonstop and was always thrilled to see him. For me, sometimes the parties evolved into too much and I would leave. Often Grandma Patty's voice rang in my head, telling me there were plenty of fish in the sea! She wanted me to find someone who would treat me right, and so did I.

I enjoyed getting to know John, but I wasn't looking for anything serious. I was adamant about that. But it's funny how things change and life surprises you. The unexpected can happen at any time.

4

The Unexpected

ON AN UNUSUALLY WARM SPRING night in early April, Liz and I jumped in my car and headed over to John's house in the heart of town. As we passed charming little shops, old architecture, landmarks, and beautiful homes, I realized how infrequently I drove into town like this.

When we arrived, we parked along the street and strolled across to his townhouse. The road was dimly lit, empty, and quiet, and the stars twinkled and shimmered in the night sky. The only sounds were the clicking of our heels on the pavement and the crickets calling from the surrounding yards.

As we approached his house, we spotted Luca and John in the alley. Upon noticing John standing there in his ripped jeans, orange sweatshirt, and backward hat, I felt my heart skip. His expansive shoulders and wide stance welcomed me in; his messy blond locks reminded me to never take life too seriously. I stopped a few feet from him, and he smiled at me. I could feel something strong between us.

I stood there, shifting my weight as I pushed my hair behind an ear and fumbled for words. Intense feelings consumed me, scaring and thrilling me all at once. I was happy to see him, and there was no denying our connection, but I wasn't looking for a boyfriend.

When I thought of John, however, I felt this magnetic pull and realized I desired to see him whenever I could. I knew in my gut that he felt it too as he kept inviting us to return. If schoolwork prevented us from getting together, I could hear the disappointment in his voice. He was quite sweet and different from other guys I had met.

After that night, John and I started to hang out one-on-one. While we were hitting it off, Liz and Luca fizzled out. It wasn't long before I made the decision to stop casually dating and began exclusively dating John. There was something special about him, and I wanted to see where it went. I threw caution to the wind and followed my heart. I began going over to his place alone to watch movies and snuggle on the couch. He had an impressive movie collection so there were plenty of titles to choose from.

John insisted on taking me on a proper date and invited me to dinner. He suggested I dress up as he was taking me someplace fancy that required that sort of attire. John was sweet, caring, and considerate, and I couldn't get enough of him and those tousled blond locks. It looked good on him, and he pulled it off. One of my favorite things about him was that he didn't care what people thought; he was always himself. He possessed a great sense of humor, and we always laughed when we were together. The hair, biceps, blue eyes, and kind smile were enough to make a girl swoon! We grew close rather quickly, and the rest was history!

Two and a half years later, we married.

5

A Beautiful but Rocky Beginning

JOHN AND I HAD A gorgeous wedding on a crisp fall day. The leaves were beginning to change and adorn the world with explosions of vibrant colors. I wore a long white dress with cranberry accents and a stunning cranberry-colored train. When I walked down the aisle that day, everything faded away except for John who stood at the altar. As we said our vows, I squeezed his hands tightly, and he smiled at me. It took me back to the day I saw him standing in the alley with that same great smile. It was the start of something beautiful.

After being married for just a few weeks, a dark cloud settled over our new life. Our world began slowly fading from vibrant autumn colors to a bleak gray. With each passing day, I experienced an increase in peculiar health issues that could not be explained.

At first, I noticed unusual reactions to food and alcohol, particularly when eating out at restaurants. Halfway through a meal, sitting at a table with family and friends, I would come close to blacking out. Dizziness and heart palpitations would take over my body, making it impossible to focus. My vision would begin to tunnel, and the voices of those around me would slow. Achy joints and hot flashes washed over me.

My only recourse was to step outside, sit on the curb for some fresh air, and let time pass. I found myself sitting on a curb alone too many times. Eating out with others became embarrassing as my reactions grew increasingly difficult to explain. Not one person seemed to comprehend how intense these sensations were or believe they were associated with something physical. Despite not living inside my body, most people were convinced I had anxiety. I was perplexed by the assumptions and opinions of others. This was going on inside *my* body, so why did they not take *my* word? Why not listen to the person living through the pain and discomfort?

When wine tasting with friends or indulging in social drinking, the same symptoms would occur. In the beginning, I thought I had lost my tolerance for alcohol. I had gotten older and wasn't partaking as often. I learned that wasn't the case when I became symptomatic regardless of where I was or what I was doing. When I was around coworkers or individuals I didn't know well, I tried to hide my issues as best I could. Feeling like I was dying inside, I pasted a smile on my face and nodded my head. In reality, I was so disoriented that I didn't know what was going on. It got harder to pretend everything was okay when my issues became more prominent and more frequent.

As I sat with my primary care doctor, nervously playing with my hair, I asked her what she thought this could be. She believed I had picked up a parasite while on my honeymoon in Aruba. It saddened me to think that something negative may have come from our honeymoon, as that trip had been such a memorable and beautiful experience.

The magnificent island of Aruba had possessed endless things to see and do. We scheduled a few activities both on and off the resort and spent the rest of our days relaxing and enjoying the amenities. Much of our time was spent with a drink in hand as we floated near the pool's swim-up bar or in a chair by the ocean.

It was my first time visiting a tropical island, and the clear blue water was breathtaking. Surrounded by sand and water, lined with palm trees that danced in the tropical breeze, I lay in the arms of my husband, taking in the sights and sounds. Soothing tunes, laughter, and joy drifted from the pool bar at a distance. With so many little nooks and cozy areas for relaxation, couples were scattered throughout. They lay in hammocks, on towels, in canopy beds draped in white linens overlooking the ocean, in beautifully designed gazebos adorned with an array of colorful flowers, on benches, under umbrellas, or among the outdoor games such as standing checkers.

Aruba stayed true to its reputation of being hot and humid, exposing me to a new climate as well as new food. After about two days into the trip, I began to experience peculiar symptoms. The first one occurred away from the resort.

We decided to go into town to check out the local shopping. The easiest way to get there was by taxi as the hotel had a constant flow of them ready to take travelers to various island locations. Outside the resort was a line of available taxis. We walked toward the first one and quickly realized these were not average-sized vehicles. John and I squeezed into the back of the tiny car, which was no larger than a MINI. I barely got the door closed before the taxi driver took off.

The roads were narrow and winding, and our driver whipped around town like Ricky Rudd in a NASCAR Road race. I guess time was money, and he wanted to cut us loose as quickly as possible so he could pick up another customer. I gripped the door tightly and leaned into every turn. This was the only way to do it or risk being tossed around like a rag doll in the back seat.

Finally, the taxi came to an abrupt halt. Thankful to have finally arrived, we exited the taxi and walked toward the mall. John and I exchanged confused glances about what had just occurred, but our attention quickly turned to the abundance of interesting shops that called out for us to explore. Stylish purses, clothing, shoes, crafts, electronics, and a variety of incredible items filled the shop windows. Possessing multiple floors, impressive architecture, and glass elevators, the mall was a treasure trove of merchandise.

We strolled around, taking in the sights of the beautiful buildings and browsing various little shops. After enjoying our time for a while, I needed a restroom break! John and I located a public bathroom, and he held my bags as I went in. The restroom was not as nice as the shops, and it was crowded. A constant stream of people came and went.

I entered a stall after waiting my turn and closed the door behind me. As I bent my legs to sit and use the toilet, I felt the ground move beneath my feet. I nearly fell over. Grabbing the wall with one hand, I braced myself. With my shorts still down at my ankles, I stood up and looked straight ahead to shake the feeling. Had the ground just moved?

I bent my legs again to sit, and the earth shifted so quickly that I collapsed into the wall. *Okay, what is going on?* I stood still and observed my surroundings. The restroom remained crowded, and I heard the voices and noises of people coming and going. No one was reacting or acting any differently and the room was still.

Is it me?

Is something wrong with me?

I closed my eyes tightly and sat on the toilet as fast as I could. I used the restroom and then slowly opened my eyes. It felt like I was swaying back and forth. Not knowing a single soul on the island, I wasn't about to ask a stranger for help. There was no cell phone reception, so texting John was out of the question. I gradually stood up while bracing myself on the wall with one hand and pulling my pants up with the other. I felt the ground move again. Over and over, the floor bucked and rolled beneath my feet as if I were on a boat floating in the ocean. Shuffling my feet, I slowly exited the stall, washed my hands, and left.

I teetered over to John who was leaning against the wall of the building.

"John! Do islands move? I mean, I know they don't... but this one is moving, so I need to be certain."

Perplexed, he responded, "No, islands don't move. Why, what's going on?"

"I feel off balance. It literally feels like this island is moving or that I'm on a boat. Every time I tried to use the restroom, the ground moved, and I fell into the wall of the stall."

"Maybe we should get you out of the sun and back to the hotel room."

I agreed. We headed back to the room and rested in the air conditioning. The cool air felt so refreshing.

I wish I could say it ended there, but it only got worse. As I sat by the pool the next afternoon, a large red rash developed on my thighs and stomach. Covering a large area, it contained tiny bumps and round edges as if taking the shape of several overlapping ovals. Immense fatigue, dizziness, and confusion accompanied the rash.

What concerned me the most about this incident was the confusion and the thick brain fog. As the fog set in, it softened and blurred the edges of everything around me. I became unable to focus and was no longer aware of what was happening. The fog was so dense and heavy that it clouded my thoughts and ability to form clear sentences. After about an hour of rest in the hotel room, the symptoms began to subside.

The next night, John and I prepared to go to the resort's Mexican restaurant for dinner. Garbed in a stunning low-cut red dress with a slit up one side to the upper thigh, I felt beautiful and bold. Red lipstick titivated my lips as did a gold choker at my neck. I had curled my dark brown hair so it bounced just below my shoulders.

The hostess led us to a corner table with dim lighting, the perfect romantic spot. Music played softly throughout the restaurant, and the tables were decorated with flickering candles and red flower petals. John held my hand across the table.

Within minutes, I was overcome with nausea and fatigue. The nausea was so intense that I was forced to excuse myself and step outside for some fresh air. Stumbling along the concrete walkway, I sat down hard on a bench that faced the main pool of the resort which was now closed. I stared at the blue water and took deep breaths through my nose and exhaled through my mouth. I closed my eyes and imagined I was somewhere else. None of it was helping. Feeling weak and frail, my vision became blurry and my body limp.

I felt a hand on my shoulder. "Kristin? Babe?"

I couldn't respond. Everything was dark.

"Babe? Are you okay?"

Colors began to reappear as my vision slowly returned.

John was standing over me, his eyes wide with fear.

"Yeah?" The susurration of my voice trailed off with the wind.

John sat beside me and pulled me into him. "Are you okay?"

"I think so… I don't know," I said quietly.

"It seems we're skipping dinner tonight. We should head back to the room."

I obliged and left feeling disappointed, guilty, and distraught about the loss of the evening.

All I could think about was how I had abandoned my husband at the dinner table on our honeymoon. I spent the rest of the night in bed attempting to recover.

Luckily, despite all the concerning health episodes, we thoroughly enjoyed each other's company and made lasting memories! I delighted in the opportunities to wear all my bridal outfits, alluring dresses, and bathing suits and loved the time spent lounging by the pool and ocean with my new husband. We had endless adventures, including a captivating experience at a butterfly farm.

As we entered the farm, butterflies enveloped us like a night sky of fireflies. Several settled on our shoulders as we strolled through the abundance of wonder. It was a pleasure to watch butterflies of various colors and sizes pause for a few moments and then flit away through the farm, creating an array of colors.

We relished the scrumptious food in Aruba. Throughout the trip, I felt as if I ate like a queen. The resort had a variety of restaurants, and each night we were able to select a different one for evening dining. Every restaurant possessed a unique environment and cuisine to create an assortment of experiences for tourists. Our favorites were the Italian restaurant and the steakhouse that overlooked the water. We could not get enough of the Italian bread dipped in olive oil and vinegar! The bread was crispy on the outside and soft and fluffy on the inside. Each dip into the seasoned balsamic vinegar mixture was heavenly. It was a struggle not to fill up on bread before the meal arrived. At the steakhouse, the steak was cooked to perfection and served alongside a picturesque view that we never wanted to leave.

We enjoyed many romantic dinners, played the slots at the resort's casino, took in a show at night, and played large checkers on the beach. We even pet iguanas that sat by the pool! We genuinely enjoyed ourselves and made some wonderful memories as a newly married couple.

6

These Are Merely Panic Attacks

AFTER OUR HONEYMOON, THINGS TURNED dark. Each day it became more challenging to get up in the morning and dress myself for work. Relentless fatigue consumed me, and persistent anxiety tortured me. Determined to maintain employment, I showed up every day and sat at my desk. Plagued with rolling panic attacks and unable to concentrate, our Employee Assistance Program (EAP) counselor became my savior. I spent half of my working days in his office, or at least it felt like I did. At each visit, he provided me with the tools to get through the panic attacks. It was my first experience with breathing exercises and meditation, which were truly the only things that got me through the day. I felt forever grateful for this man and knew I would never forget how he helped me.

My primary care doctor's first potential diagnosis was parasites. With my recent visit out of the country, it seemed logical. Nervous and distressed by my decline in health, I tried to hold onto the memories of our unforgettable honeymoon and remain positive. John and I vowed to move forward and to figure this out together.

When the blood work came back negative, we were surprised. Of course, it was good news, but it also meant we had to explore other potential causes.

As time passed, my health further deteriorated. Dizziness and an off-balance feeling made mobility difficult. The more I pushed myself to act "normal," the worse I got. My body became a constant distraction and hindrance, feeling heavy and somnolent throughout the day. At night, I sat in a warm bath to soothe my aching joints and muscles, the weight of unfinished chores and responsibilities on my shoulders. I continued to return to my primary care physician, but she was perplexed and at a loss for what might be causing the symptoms. She suspected hypoglycemia, but as I worsened, she insisted it was anxiety and panic. Convinced this had to be the answer, she prescribed benzos (Benzodiazepines) and SSRIs (Selective Serotonin Reuptake Inhibitors). Desperate to feel better, I took the medications even though I didn't agree with the diagnosis.

I should have listened to my inner voice, which was telling me that it was not anxiety. Instead, I began to doubt myself and trust the doctor. I made peace with the fact that anxiety and panic may be the cause. Maybe I was stressed at my new job, with getting married, purchasing a home, or graduating from college. I had experienced several life-changing events back to back. Perhaps I was tired and stressed. I probably was.

But all the changes in my life had been positive ones, and I had been young and healthy. My gut told me that something else was wrong. It felt like much more. However, based on the recommendation of my doctor, I went ahead and took an SSRI called Lexapro and a benzo named Klonopin. I was quite desperate for help, so I put my trust in my doctor instead of my instinct.

Two weeks later, I began to feel worse. My moods were unpredictable: one minute I was crying, the next I was elated, and then hours later, I didn't want to live anymore. I stayed in a state of panic with an erratic heart rate and a fight-or-flight response that remained perpetually activated.

My body was in a state of disarray and there was no off switch to be found. Not a moment went by where I couldn't feel my own heart beating in my chest. It was a constant *thump thump, thump thump* and would flutter high up into my throat. The feeling of being on a boat stuck out at sea persisted as the ground continued to move beneath my feet. *Why was this happening?*

I called my primary care doctor, and they assured me I was experiencing panic attacks that would pass. These panic attacks became merciless and recurrent. I was miserable. Rocking back and forth at my desk, I pulled at my hair and fidgeted with my favorite pen. The sound of the nearby door opening and closing grew louder and louder, and the cold air drafting in went right through my bones. I shivered and bounced my leg up and down as I stared at my computer screen. The screen was full of words I was required to read but there was no way I could focus. My mind was full of irrational thoughts and chaos; there was no room for anything else.

Trying to fight off the thoughts, I sat at my desk as long as I could tolerate. It was a struggle to stay warm and impossible to get any work done. I continued to visit the EAP counselor to survive. I became completely unable to make it through a workday without having the counselor talk me through these violent attacks. It was clear to me that I needed help with these new intense symptoms. I called my doctor's office repeatedly in an attempt to reach them. Each week, I was brushed off by the staff until one day the nurse finally put my doctor on the phone.

"Hello, how can I help you today?" Dr. Blossom asked.

"Dr. Blossom, something is wrong. My heart is racing and no matter what I do, I can't get it to stop. I'm feeling dizzy all the time. My moods are a mess. I just don't know what to do."

"Kristin, I've told you before—these are *merely* panic attacks. You need to ride them out. I don't know what else to tell you."

"Are you sure?" I asked.

"Yes, I'm sure. It's the only thing that makes sense," replied Dr. Blossom.

"I don't think that anxiety is my problem. I still feel sick, and now I just feel worse," I said.

"I don't know what to tell you. I don't think I can help you anymore," said Dr. Blossom.

"What do you mean?" I asked.

Dr. Blossom began to yell through the phone, "Kristin, I told you already that you have anxiety and panic attacks! I don't know how to help you anymore! I think it's time for you to stop calling here and find a new practice!" She hung up.

I was in shock. Had my doctor, a medical professional, actually just yelled at me and hung up? I was calling her out of desperation and searching for answers, and she was unwilling to be my partner in that search. It was then that I realized something: she didn't know *how* to help me. She didn't *understand* what was going on and she was *giving up*. Dr. Blossom couldn't fight for me.

Perhaps she had gotten frustrated with herself and her lack of knowledge and taken it out on me. Had she really thought I simply had anxiety and panic? And even if that were the case, why would she have so apathetically described them as "mere" panic attacks? I was angered beyond belief. She had invalidated my struggles, implying that panic attacks were no big deal when, in fact, they are a horrific experience for anyone who suffers through them. They were much worse because of the medication *she* put me on. I didn't know for sure what was going on except that she clearly wasn't the doctor for me.

One week later, I ended up in the hospital with unbearable dizziness and repeat syncopal (loss of consciousness) episodes. I was now a professional at blacking out and could anticipate almost every occurrence. As an episode arose, my entire body tingled and grew hot, and the edges of my vision would soften, tunneling into a black hole. As soon as I felt the tingling, I would shout out to those around me to prepare them in case I injured myself during the fall. Each episode happened so quickly that I often wondered how loud my shouting actually was. It was hard to distinguish reality from the dreamlike state that enveloped me.

Fainting was not my only issue as I suffered from unpredictable moods which troubled everyone I encountered. Violent outbursts of anger, sadness, fear, and pure jubilation would surface at any time. Such emotional whiplash had led me to contemplate crashing my vehicle into my doctor's office.

I lay in a hospital bed, once again in the gown I loved so much. Looking around at the four walls of my room and taking in the familiar hospital smell, my eyes met the whiteboard to the left of me.

What level is your pain?

It went from no pain (a green smiley face) to the worst pain possible (a red smiley face). These options felt very inadequate as if a green or red smiley face could describe what I was going through.

"Good afternoon, Kristin." My thoughts were interrupted by the doctor abruptly entering the room.

"Hello, Doctor."

"So, tell me, what's been going on with you? What brings you here today?"

I did my best to collect my thoughts and began describing my mood changes, heart palpitations, syncope, hives, food reactions, lack of energy, and the pain I had been experiencing.

"It seems you are having difficulty with this medication, and it appears to have made you manic. We need to get you tapered off it immediately. I don't think it's beneficial."

I couldn't believe my ears! Someone was listening. I had an answer to my new symptoms. The medication was making me manic. I had never been on medication like this before.

"Really?"

"Yes. I'd like you to begin tapering off the medication and follow up with your primary care doctor."

Discontinuing the medication was welcome advice—I was happy with this as I hadn't thought it was the right option in the first place. Seeing my primary care doctor, however, I would not do. I had to find someone new.

I lay in bed that night exhausted and drained. After the hospital discharged me, it was nice to be back home in my bed with John.

"It will be okay," said John. "We will figure this out. At least we know now that the medication was not the right choice for you."

"Yeah, that's true," I said.

"I never thought it was solely anxiety anyway. There is something much bigger going on with you. I wish somebody would figure it out."

"God, I hope so. I don't know how much more of this I can take."

We were then interrupted by the ringing of my cell phone. It was my mom, Meg. I had already received text messages from a few friends including Liz. I appreciated it when friends and family checked in on me after something like this. It's always nice to know someone cares.

"Hey, Mom."

"Hey, are you home now?"

"Yeah, I'm lying in bed."

"So, how are you? What did the hospital say?"

"I'm okay. Just tired. They said the medication was making me manic and to begin tapering off of it."

"Wow, really?"

"Yup."

"What do you think?"

"It makes sense. I haven't felt right since I got on the medication. I've gotten worse and not better."

"Well, I hope you feel better soon. I won't keep you. Get some rest tonight. Call me tomorrow."

"Okay, I will."

I hung up. John must have noticed how stressed I seemed.

"Come here, babe," he said.

He put his arm around me, and I lay on his chest. After such a long, taxing night, John's arms felt just right. This was the only place I wanted to be—in the arms of the man I love.

7

Your Blood Work Is Normal

LIFE WAS BLEAK. JOINT PAIN, tingling and numbness in my extremities, syncope, dizziness, debilitating fatigue, calf and foot pain, and brain fog riddled my mind and body. The most prominent symptom was intense pain in my lower right abdomen; it kept me up night after night. I lay awake, tossing and turning wondering when the agony would end. My insides twisted into a tight knot, followed by the sheer pain of a sharp blade. There was nothing I could do to remove this blade from my body. The pain was relentless, never allowing me to come up for air. I quickly tired with no relief in sight. It was time to search for another doctor.

Based on the recommendations of others, I was able to locate a new doctor and was willing to give her a shot. I scheduled my first appointment. *Here goes nothing*, I thought with little optimism.

The new doctor immediately rattled off various tests to order and explained that pain in that particular area could be indicative of a cyst.

It felt more like deep muscle pain to me, and a cyst seemed unlikely. But, once again, I allowed her to run the blood work. It was worth checking to rule it out. I was hopeful, but not convinced.

My gut instinct was right again. The blood work found nothing, the doctor found nothing wrong, and I ended up leaving that practice as well. That visit took me along another path that eventually led to a dead end. The only suggestion provided to me was to take Advil every six hours for the pain in my abdomen. Advil covers up pain and does not determine the root cause. It was not a permanent solution and repeated use of NSAIDs can cause problems. I felt discouraged.

Still with no answers and nowhere to turn, my health remained poor. My absences from work became more frequent, and my quality of life deteriorated. Visits to the hospital increased, as did referrals to specialists. My life was now consumed with endless doctor visits and medical testing. I became numb to the idea of being stuck with a needle and would hold out my arm without batting an eye. IVs and blood work were like brushing my teeth—part of my routine. It felt like the smell of the hospital was permanently engrained in my skin. I couldn't wash it off. I was tired. I was sick. I was confused. Each doctor I saw was stumped.

This seems to be the way most Lyme stories, and many other chronic illnesses, begin. Slowly, your health starts to fade, and you begin to lose yourself. Visits to the doctor move to the forefront of your life and begin to take over. Doctor after doctor is unable to discover anything significant and they tell you that nothing is wrong. They tell you it is all in your head, and sometimes you believe them.

"Have you been feeling stressed lately?"

"Your blood work looks normal. I see nothing wrong."

"It's probably hormones."

"It's anxiety. Have you tried (insert SSRI drug here)?"

"You are having a panic attack."

"You need more rest."

"Have you seen a therapist?"

Sound familiar to anyone? These sorts of responses confuse the patient, and they second-guess themselves. Unable to understand why these symptoms are occurring, they stop listening to their gut and start to believe that maybe the doctors are right, that maybe they should try this drug or that drug—whichever drug the doctor pushes their way, hoping it will solve the issue and the patient will leave their office. Many doctors throw darts at the problem and apply band-aids without uncovering any real solutions.

When I was told I was experiencing anxiety and panic, I thought, *Of course I'm having a panic attack! I passed out yesterday and my body is in a state of crisis. I am no longer able to complete basic tasks such as sweeping the house and my relationship with my new husband is suffering. My*

friends are slipping away. My job is slipping away. My life is slipping away.
My mind is struggling, and my body is hurting. That would give anyone anxiety!

I was sick and nobody could figure out why! Anxiety and panic are a chicken and egg situation: is the anxiety a symptom of a medical condition, or does the medical condition bring on the anxiety? Doctors don't talk about this enough. Patients are regularly blamed for their mental state when, in fact, the culprit could be a medical issue.

Innumerable specialists examined me, each searching for a cause. None found an answer. I knew in my heart that it was not solely anxiety. Multiple organ systems do not deteriorate and become symptomatic from anxiety alone. These symptoms were causing regular visits to the Emergency Department, and I was growing weary of it. Something was wrong with my body, and it was affecting my mental health and my life. Often, it felt like the relatively healthy life I had lived prior was something in the far-off distance. A memory of a past life.

8

You Must Be Anorexic

ONCE AGAIN, I FOUND MYSELF in a hospital bed: sick, weak, frail, and in pain. My stomach was wrecked, and my joints were aching. Plagued with ruthless stomach pain, repeated visits to the bathroom, syncope, dehydration, and stiff inflamed joints, I was tortured inside my own body. At this point, I weighed less than eighty-five pounds and was desperate for nutrition and a solution. I had been continuously poked and prodded only to get nowhere. Prior to this visit, a gastroenterologist performed an endoscopy to investigate stomach concerns. Not only did the test find nothing, but I awoke during the procedure. I can vividly remember feeling the tube in my throat, but being unable to speak and express my fear and discomfort.

As my feeble body existed in my hospital room, my thoughts trailed off imagining I was someplace else. In my mind, I could be anything and be anywhere. Full of energy, carefree, and able to travel and see the world. I could stand on the streets of Paris, surrounded by architectural landmarks, beautiful gardens, and stunning sophistication. It was nothing but pure elegance and beauty. I had never truly been to Paris, but my friend, Malorie, had shared her recent photos with me and they burned images into my brain.

The nurse entered my room, jolting my thoughts back to the present. She expressed that an endocrinologist would be joining me shortly as the ER doctor suspected problems with my thyroid. *Yet another doctor thrown at my problems. I wonder where this dart will land.*

What happened next was so unexpected, it would leave me feeling rattled and disparaged. Simultaneously, the endocrinologist

29

and nurse grew combative and inquired whether I was anorexic. Grilling me about what I had eaten that day, they belittled and berated me until I felt small, decrepit, and alone. The line of questioning felt like an interrogation and was not inquisitive or empathetic. I feebly muttered responses, explaining that I did not have anorexia, but that eating created visits to the bathroom due to diarrhea. I ate, but my body rejected it. Dismissive, they acted as if I were a burden and possessed zero desire to help me. I was left shocked by the poor treatment I received and the abuse I endured as a patient that day in the hospital. Defeated, I reached my breaking point.

I wondered how I would go on, feeling like a lab rat and an experiment and not treated as a person by the medical community. I was looked at as a problem, one they didn't want to deal with. The treatment I received only worsened my pain and suffering. I was dismissed, abused, ignored, and left to feel completely abandoned. Misunderstood and seen as too complicated, I was gaslit by doctors who were unable to identify the problem, insisting it was all in my head.

On top of the acute struggles of my medical condition, my life was falling apart. I continually brooded about the potential of losing my marriage or my career. It was at that moment that I began to see doctors as humans with flaws who, at times, lacked knowledge, compassion, or understanding. They don't always have the answers, and they may not want to admit that. Not every human is capable of admitting when they are wrong or when they don't have the answers. My faith in the medical community slipped away, just like my health.

As all these feelings swirled around in my head, my own thoughts became louder and louder and an anger grew inside me. I cracked. As I struggled to sit up, weak and fragile in my hospital bed, I suddenly began to yell and swear out loud. My brittle body looked like a stick inside the hospital gown, and my face was red with anger. A fire of uncontrollable obscenities spewed from my mouth like a dragon.

Completely consumed with anger and frustration, I gave the doctor no chance to speak or respond. As soon as the doctor left the room, I looked at John and continued to scream, "That doctor is a complete asshole! He better never fucking return to my room! Keep him the hell out of my sight! I can't believe the nerve of that guy! Anorexic? I would kill for a good meal if I could keep anything down and it didn't rip through my stomach like an explosion! Un-fucking-believable!"

John just looked at me, unsure of what to say or do. He was angry too; I could see it on his face. He listened and agreed and then began to pace the room with his lips pursed together in anger. I could tell he was trying to hold it together.

"I know, babe. They were bad today. Why would they assume it is anorexia? Obviously, you're sick. You wouldn't have checked yourself into the hospital looking for answers if that weren't the case. Who the fuck does he think he is? Oh, here is a small girl getting even smaller—she must be anorexic. What the fuck? Yeah, buddy, the solution is to eat more! You've cracked the case! Holy shit, you've done it!"

Our anger and disappointment weren't going to help anything. Yelling used up any strength I had left to give for the night. I was too tired to put any more thought or energy into being angry or upset.

9

I Felt Normal, Maybe Even Free

AFTER THAT DELIGHTFUL AND INSPIRING hospital experience, I followed up with a different endocrinologist. He ordered blood work, conducted tests, diagnosed me with potential pre-diabetes, and prescribed yet another drug for me to take. I continued to feel like a rat in a lab as doctors diagnosed me with various ailments and prescribed a cocktail of drugs. I discovered how quickly doctors jumped to prescribing pharmaceuticals for treatment, sometimes even when they were not confident in their diagnosis.

I decided I wasn't going to take the prescription. This doctor did not seem confident in his diagnosis as he even used the word "potential." I wasn't about to put my body through another drug until I knew a diagnosis was certain or there was at least a clear indication that it could be helpful. Why were we jumping straight to drugs and not discussing diet and other natural solutions? Why were we not trying to identify the root cause?

I needed some time away from doctors to feel like a human being again. I was spending most of my time in bed or at a doctor's office. When I could, I would drag myself to work. That task alone was a feat. Walking to my desk took an eternity as I struggled to maintain balance and energy. The long endless hallway that led to my desk seemed to extend farther with every attempt. Each time I took a step, my knee joints felt like creaky old doors trying to break loose of the hinges.

After my appointment, John and I decided to get out of the house and go for a drive. I wanted to spend some time in nature and feel the cool breeze in my hair and the warm sun on my face. We decided to drive to a local historic home and garden known for its beauty. When we arrived, John helped me out of the car. I stepped out onto the gravel parking area on my shaky legs. He grabbed my hand and held it in his and put his arm around me. We walked around a bit through the seven acres of gardens and the beautiful landscape. We took a stroll down a small path into a beautiful meadow, which led us past a pond and a water garden.

"I need to take a break," I said. I could feel my body becoming weaker and weaker. I adored the scenery, but I could walk no farther. My body was hunched over; my pace had slowed to a dawdling trudge.

"Okay, let's sit right here near this pond. Wow, look at all the fish!" exclaimed John.

John had always been mesmerized by fish. When we met, he had owned a fish tank in his townhouse. During cold winter months, he liked to go to the pet store and look at the fish in the aquariums. During the warm seasons, he enjoyed fishing anywhere he could.

John tossed down a blanket and helped me sit by the pond so I could enjoy the scenery. I loved the look and sound of the nearby water fountain. The water was clear as glass, trickling down from the top of the fountain and splashing to the bottom. It was the focal point of the garden, and its sound was incredibly relaxing.

I closed my eyes and let my mind drift away with the rhythmic pitter-patter, allowing me to feel as if I were totally alone among the mellifluous melody. I stretched out on the blanket, arched my back, and turned toward the sun.

A cool breeze tugged at my hair and cooled my heated skin. The sun was warm enough that I could feel it on my face. I never wanted to leave this place. It was the most relaxed I had felt in months. In the calm and special quality of nature, I felt normal, maybe even free.

10

Click My Heels Three Times

BUT I WAS SOON YANKED back to reality. If I wanted to get better, I couldn't avoid doctors forever. I just needed to find the right one.

I had high hopes for my next doctor's appointment as the facility had an excellent reputation. It was a referral to the University of Virginia Medical Center.

John and I drove to Charlottesville, Virginia, and booked a hotel room for the night before the appointment. My depleted body found traveling difficult because it increased my stress and changed my routine. I quickly learned this trip would be no different as we arrived at the hotel.

Standing at the check-in counter, I leaned against John for support. A woman with dark hair sporting wisps of gray sat behind the counter. She hunched over in her chair and wrinkled her nose as she typed at her computer. Banging the keys, her face scowled and her nostrils flared. John and I waited a few minutes, but she never acknowledged our presence.

John began shifting his weight and let out a sigh. "Hello. Excuse me, would you mind checking us in?"

Without looking up, the woman replied, "Name?"

John gave her the information, and she continued typing.

"You'll be in room 407," she murmured. "Take the elevator up to the fourth floor and then take an immediate left. Have a nice stay." With that, she waved her hand as if to swat us away like flies.

John thanked her, and we made our way upstairs.

"Boy, she was friendly," he remarked. I smiled at him as we entered the elevator. The ride was short, but I wanted it to end. I held onto him as the elevator ascended. My body was crashing; I could feel it. All I wanted to do was lie down and get off my trembling legs.

As we reached the fourth floor, the elevator doors opened and we stepped out onto a dark blue, patterned carpet. Taking an immediate left, we followed the long hall toward our room. Almost immediately, I felt my heart rate increase and the dizziness kick in. Unsteady on my feet and relying heavily on John, I knew this was a bad sign. Whenever my heart acted this badly, it was relentless and did not improve without intervention. With John's support, I managed to make it to our hotel bed to lie down. By this point, my heart was furiously hammering like an offbeat orchestra. Who was conducting this thing?

I remained in bed for a while, but the symptoms did not subside.

"John, I still don't feel well and it's not letting up. I don't know what's wrong with me. If I stand up, I might pass out again."

"Maybe we should take you to the hospital."

"Oh, God, the hospital? Again? I don't want to go."

"I know, but what other option is there?"

"Maybe we should wait until my appointment in the morning. We've been here less than an hour. What about the room?"

"Don't worry about the room. How about I get you some salt water? Let's see if that helps you feel better."

"Okay, that sounds good." Salt water had proved to be beneficial in the past, so I liked that idea.

John left and came back with a cold bottle of water. He reached into my purse for a salt packet, ripped it open, and poured it into the water bottle. He gave it a good shake and then passed the unusual beverage to me. I sipped it while I lay in bed.

"I feel like I'm going to throw up now. I don't think it's getting any better."

"Okay, that's it. We are going to the hospital," declared John.

I nodded in agreement. I didn't want to go, but being so far away from home, there were not many options.

With our arms interlocked for balance, we headed back down to the front desk. John's face was wrinkled with worry as he watched me struggle. Pale and unable to stand, I tried my best to hold it together and not faint.

John was ready for the unfriendly desk clerk this time. Sternly, he explained that we needed to leave immediately and head over to the hospital. I hoped we would be able to get a refund, especially with all the money we spent on medical appointments. With every doctor visit, I watched as our hard-earned money vanished into a black hole. Our bank account was draining at a dangerous rate. Luckily, the hotel provided us a refund, (but gave us a hard time about it), and we headed over to the UVA Hospital emergency room.

Upon arrival at the facility, a nurse came to take my vitals and ask questions. Due to my cardiovascular symptoms, I was abruptly placed in a wheelchair and taken back to the triage area. The unfamiliar and eerie environment made me uneasy. I wished I was home or at least at my local hospital.

Wheeling toward triage, I was surprised at what I saw. It was a large space comprised of three walls divided using thin blue curtains for privacy. The front was open to a hallway full of nurses and staff. I was placed in the last divided space at the end, which had a blue curtain on each side. It was setup and run differently than what I was used to, and the ER was chaotic with very little privacy.

From behind the curtain diagonally across from me, I heard the raspy voice of an older raucous gentleman. "I've been drugged, I tell ya! Did you hear what I said? Drugged. I'm pissin' blood. Did you hear me? Drugged. Be careful, ma'am."

Just as he finished his sentence, I heard vomit splash onto the floor and saw the nurse jump back. The curtain didn't quite reach the ground so I could see her feet scurrying about the area. He then began to cough repeatedly and forcefully. It sounded painful.

"You're bleeding, sir. Let me get you cleaned up," said the nurse.

"Bleeding? Where?" the man asked.

"From your mouth, sir," replied the nurse.

"Shit! I told you they drugged me!" gagged the man.

What the hell was going on over there? I felt dirty and grossed out. I wanted to crawl out of my skin and leave my body that was

36

failing me. Uncomfortable, sick, and in agony, I wished I was somewhere else. I was nauseous and on the verge of vomiting, and this environment was not quelling that. I thought of Dorothy in the *Wizard of Oz*, wishing I could click my heels three times and be elsewhere.

A trip to the ER is distressing, especially on a hectic night. It can be unpredictable, and you never know if it will be a positive or negative experience.

Eventually, I was removed from triage and given a room. Thankful for a little privacy and quiet, I felt my body release some tension. This was much better, but not nearly as nice as my local hospital. The room smelled sour and damp and appeared unclean and unorganized. All hospitals have that "hospital smell," but this was different. There was a foul-smelling odor, and blood spots misted the wall. After every hospital visit, I couldn't wait to take a shower. I could already sense that tonight my desire for a shower would be stronger than usual.

The doctor and nurses administered IV fluids and monitored my heart rate. After two bags of fluids, I felt a sense of relief and calm. As my heart began to feel better, I put two and two together: IV fluids were immensely helpful. This stuff was like gold for my body!

We spent all night in the ER and were told to follow up with the UVA diabetes and endocrinology doctor in the morning. They were unsure of the cause of my symptoms but felt confident the doctor could help me at my appointment. With zero sleep, we went straight from the hospital to the doctor's office. Sitting in the waiting room, bleary-eyed, we talked about what a long and stressful night it had been. I didn't get the shower that I desperately wanted and was wearing the clothes from the day before. Burned in my nostrils was the scent of isopropyl alcohol mixed with the foul-smelling mystery odor.

The only thing I looked forward to was the possibility that Dr. Lewis would have some good news or thoughts to share. I hoped my visit would prove to be worth it.

Once we were in the exam room, we surprisingly didn't have to wait long for the doctor to come in. Dr. Lewis was in his mid-sixties and boasted salt-and-pepper hair, wire-rimmed glasses, and nets of wrinkles at the corner of his eyes. He towered over me as he smiled and introduced himself.

"Hi, I'm Dr. Lewis. Nice to meet you folks today. I hear you had a long night."

"Yes, we did," I replied.

"Okay, well, let's look at your records from the hospital. Tell me what happened and what brings you here today."

I proceeded to explain my symptoms to the doctor and the events that led to my hospital visit. John jumped in and assisted as needed. I was beginning to have trouble remembering things, and John knew that. It was one of my many symptoms and it was nice to have him along to help me through it.

Dr. Lewis thought for a moment. "Okay, well, I'd like to send you home with a glucose monitor and check your blood sugar daily. Let's see if we can eliminate that as an issue. I also want you to record your symptoms in a notebook or diary and bring that with you to your next appointment. It sounds like you are having what we call a vasovagal response."

"Vasovagal? What is that?"

"We all have what's called a vagus nerve. When the nerve is irritated due to certain triggers, this can cause syncope and issues with your blood pressure and heart rate."

"Oh, wow. Okay." This was something new. I hadn't yet heard of the vagus nerve.

"So, we will provide you with the glucose monitor. You'll need to prick your finger daily using the monitor. There's a book inside that you can use to track your results. Then let's see you back in three weeks."

"Okay, sounds good," I said.

"Any questions?"

"No, I don't think so."

"Take care of yourself, all right?" he said with a smile and put his hand on my shoulder.

"Okay, thank you."

This was the first piece of information I'd received from a medical professional that made sense to me. I was having a vasovagal response potentially related to blood sugar. There could be a connection here to my first symptoms, which occurred after eating and consuming alcohol.

The doctor sent me home with a blood glucose monitor, and I began pricking my finger every day. It was another less-than-desirable experience to add to the list, but I was thankful it wasn't another drug! The idea of pricking my finger made me nervous, and I was hesitant at first. After a few days, it got easier. I did notice that the tips of my fingers started to get sore.

When I went over the readings with the doctor at my next appointment, he said my blood sugar was normal. No issues. This was good news! Still concerned about the syncope episodes, he referred me to a neurologist. I was very grateful for his knowledge, kindness, and understanding and for being the first doctor to point me in the right direction.

11

Excellent Doctors

THE MEDICAL COMMUNITY IS FULL of human beings, just like any other profession. We are all flawed and imperfect and are not always operating at our best. It's understandable and forgivable, right? We also can't possibly be expected to know it all.

But what goes beyond acceptable flaws for a doctor? What would truly be considered characteristics or behaviors of a doctor providing poor medical care? What if they are cold, dismissive, and arrogant, or have poor communication and listening skills? What if they make you feel invalidated? Forgotten? Crazy? What if their ego gets in the way and they are unable to utter the words, "I don't know?" What if they don't make attempts to prevent disease before it starts? What if by possessing all these qualities, they are causing harm to their patients?

I encountered this time and time again, and it was discouraging. I was losing faith in the medical community and found myself left with disappointment and sorrow. I was mourning the loss of something, and that was the trust I placed in their hands. It was gone now.

If it hadn't been for the excellent doctors I came across, my trust would have been lost forever. Luckily, some stepped up to the plate, and I eventually found *quality* medical care. What are the characteristics of an excellent doctor providing *quality* medical care? How would you feel if they were compassionate, investigative, listened to you, and provided collaborative care? What if you truly felt like part of a team? What if they continued their education and research, always expanding their knowledge? How would you feel then? Would you feel that they were helping you and other patients to the best of their ability? What kind of difference would it make if they were humble and empathetic instead of combative and arrogant? Would you feel relaxed and heard and ready to listen to their advice? Would you feel hopeful instead of discouraged?

That's how I felt when I finally found doctors who were willing to work with me. It brought out new passion and hope that had been taken away from me. It reignited the investigative and analytical part of my brain that wanted answers. Just as I was ready to give up, these doctors brought me back.

Before I get back into my story, it's worth discussing this issue. Providing anything less than quality medical care can be dangerous and even disastrous to a patient's physical and mental well-being, and it happens more often than it should. Doctors all over the country, and the world, are failing patients. There are several reasons for this.

The U.S. healthcare system is broken and riddled with issues that impact a doctor's ability to do their job properly. Doctors are restricted and controlled by their own administrative and hospital policies, health insurance companies, the Centers for Disease Control and Prevention (CDC), the Infectious Diseases Society of America (IDSA), and the medical training they receive. Their training has mostly been focused on acute care and has not been investigative or functional. On top of this, doctors are regularly lobbied by the deep pockets of pharmaceutical companies, which perpetuates the sick care system and continues to encourage the use of band-aid treatments. They are trained to play by the rules— which no longer serve us in today's society. The system is flawed and failing its patients.

People are growing sicker and beginning to wake up and demand better. An increase in chronic illness cases has led to the need for longer appointments. However, doctors are overwhelmed and are not compensated for lengthy appointments or for spending time conducting medical research. Mainstream medical doctors are trained to operate in a *sick* care system, not in an investigative capacity, and to push patients through utilizing fifteen-minute appointments. How much can you learn and help someone in fifteen minutes? Time with patients is what is truly needed, but it has not been made attainable due to restrictions placed on doctors.

Medical school itself can present a problem as some topics are only briefly covered on a single page, leading to a lack of knowledge or a belief that a condition must be rare. This can be one reason why a patient is passed from specialist to specialist. This creates visits with multiple doctors as well as several diagnoses and treatment plans, leading a patient to ultimately feel tossed around and hopeless.

How often do patients give up when they find themselves in this endless loop? Do they continue to seek out the medical care they need and deserve?

True hope and healing are gained when you meet a doctor who truly listens to you, finds your health problems intriguing, and possesses a desire to solve the puzzle you present. They feel empathy for how sick you are and want to help. They are concerned and can't let you leave their office until they can help in some way. They provide exploratory and preventative care versus acute care and search for root causes.

It's not just patients who are painfully aware of the flaws in the healthcare system; it's doctors too. Some have had to learn to work around the system to provide the attention patients truly deserve. This is what I would consider an excellent doctor who truly follows the Hippocratic Oath.

It's what we all deserve. It's what we all need.

The system is broken, and it needs to change.

I'm grateful that through persistence and research, I finally found a set of doctors who took this positive approach, but it should have happened much sooner. Patients shouldn't have to work so hard to locate quality care, particularly during their lowest and sickest moments.

12

A Fork in the Road

CHRONIC ILLNESS IS A LONG and grueling journey. Days are filled with struggling to survive and searching for answers that may never come. The journey requires trudging through rough terrain and dragging your body across desolate deserts and up steep mountains.

Surrounded by a landscape of sand, the harsh heat of the sun beats down on your tattered and depleted body. Finally collapsing, you find that digging your fingers into the sand helps you drag yourself along farther and farther. Your throat becomes dry, and your heart pounds faster as you search for water. Hoping to see even just a puddle, you encounter nothing but a dried-up creek.

Along the outskirts of the desert, you approach the sloping side of a steep mountain. The view is enough to destroy all hope as it appears impossible to climb. Slowly making your way up the incline, the wind howls, and strong gusts try to knock you down. Pushing against you, the gales laugh at your feeble attempts. You reach up to wipe dirt and sweat off your forehead with the back of your hand. Surprised that you have any sweat left, you lick your dry lips and feel disoriented from dehydration.

Your legs are weak. Cuts, bruises, and scrapes burn and bleed. As the sky grows dark, you hunker down for the night. Sleeping under an overhanging boulder, you shiver under the nighttime sky. Stars twinkle overhead, reminding you that the world is much bigger than yourself. Wishing for a miracle, you rest in the dirt and hope the next day will be different, that when you wake, things will be better. You will find yourself on a new path.

Each path we find ourselves on during our journey can lead to different outcomes. We are faced with many difficult decisions which force us to choose a way forward. These decisions can lead you in the right direction toward healing, hurtle you toward another mountain, or drop you at a dead end.

As I continued my journey, I arrived at a fork in the road. I stood there alone staring at my options, feeling completely frustrated and depleted. I knew I had a decision to make, but which path should I choose? John was there to support me, but in the end, I knew the decision was mine and mine alone. I agonized over which decision was best and weighed the pros and cons.

Decisions like these are never easy, especially for someone who tends to overthink. The path to the left was short and straightforward. It seemed safe, relatively risk-averse, and appeared well-worn as if it were traveled frequently. The path to the right was longer and winding. It was more difficult to see what obstacles I might encounter since the trail was overgrown with brush and ivy. I could see some brush ahead, indicating it may be less traveled. I wondered endlessly: *Which path should I take? Which one looks safest and most promising? Does one look easier than the other? If it is an easier path, is that what matters? Which path will lead me to answers and better health, both of which I am desperately seeking?*

The path to the left followed mainstream medicine and had me continuing to heed the advice of doctors. Would this path benefit me? How had that approach served me thus far? It hadn't.

This led me to the path to the right—my final decision. On this path, I would continue to fight and persist, follow my gut instinct, and go where the universe guided me. I would seek out doctors who listened and who I felt added value to my overall well-being. This decision threw me into an extremely extensive and painful but rewarding journey. I didn't realize the impact this decision would have on my life.

My first stop on this path was the office of Dr. Joy, a neurologist located in my small town. Looking back, I understand just how much I owe him for listening to me and presenting some intriguing ideas. I had traveled seeking answers, but my journey had led me right back to my own town.

My first visit with Dr. Joy was surprisingly informative. Its purpose was to follow up on my symptom of vasovagal syncope.

Asking thorough questions, he seemed genuinely interested and somewhat fascinated with the case I presented. He indicated my symptoms sounded like Postural Orthostatic Tachycardia Syndrome (POTS). When I first heard this diagnosis, I was mystified: I'd never heard of it before, and it sounded like what you put a plant in or something you smoke.

I learned that "POTS is a form of dysautonomia, a disorder of the autonomic nervous system. This branch of the nervous system regulates functions we don't consciously control, such as heart rate, blood pressure, sweating, and body temperature. The key characteristics of POTS are specific symptoms and an exaggerated increase in heart rate when standing."[2] That could explain the difficulty I had been having with my heart rate, syncope, and heat.

Dr. Joy provided information that described POTS as, "a blood circulation disorder characterized by two factors: a specific group of symptoms that frequently occur when standing upright; a heart rate increase from horizontal to standing (or as tested on a tilt table) of at least thirty beats per minute in adults, or at least forty beats per minute in adolescents, measured during the first ten minutes of standing."[3]

The symptoms of POTS can "include but are not limited to, lightheadedness (occasionally with fainting), difficulty thinking and concentrating (brain fog), fatigue, intolerance of exercise, headache, blurry vision, palpitations, tremor and nausea."[4]

Wow, I thought. *These symptoms sound familiar!* The neurologist took the time to clarify that a person doesn't just get POTS and that there must be an underlying cause. Based on my symptoms, he believed that the cause was a spirochete infection called Lyme disease. He explained that Lyme disease is caused by a corkscrew-shaped bacteria called Borrelia burgdorferi that drills into different parts of your body. Since I was presenting many symptoms, mostly neurological, it would make sense that this bacterium had already affected several organ systems. He genuinely believed I had Lyme

---

[2] "Postural Orthostatic Tachycardia Syndrome (POTS)," John Hopkins Medicine, Accessed October 17, 2023, https://www.hopkinsmedicine.org/health/conditions-and-diseases/postural-orthostatic-tachycardia-syndrome-pots?amp=true.
[3] Ibid.
[4] Ibid.

disease that had gone untreated and unfortunately caused POTS. I watched him look at me with real concern as he told me I was a very sick young woman.

By that point, I had deteriorated so drastically that I was unable to hold my head up as I sat in a chair in the exam room. My mother and the doctor pushed my chair against the wall so I could use it to prop up my head during my appointment.

Frail, thin, and still weighing under eighty-five pounds, my arms hung at my sides and my eyes were heavy with fatigue. On days like that day, I was unable to drive myself to medical appointments. My ability to transport myself had been compromised, so I drove less often.

No longer able to drive myself to medical appointments, my mother had become my ride. I was rarely driving now, and only on better days, which were infrequent, or days where I was feeling particularly stubborn.

The doctor felt strongly about Lyme disease and encouraged me to see a specialist, so I decided I would research it. For now, I would be placed on a beta blocker to treat the POTS and hope for the best. Dr. Joy looked at me with concern in his eyes and ordered that I discontinue driving altogether; he would reevaluate my ability to drive in six months.

The moment he uttered those words, profound sadness overcame me. There I was, newly married, unable to drive at twenty-four years old, and fighting for my life. I still feel truly thankful for Dr. Joy. There was something different about him and about this visit: for the first time, a doctor was listening to me and seeing my pain. I left his office with a blood work order to test for Lyme disease, as well as an order to schedule a tilt table test at the hospital.

13

What Happened to Your Face?

OPENING MY EYES EACH MORNING and feeling my body again was a constant disappointment. For some reason, I expected things to be different, but they never were. No matter how often I prayed for improvement, I remained on repeat. This day was no different.

I immediately felt exhaustion, aching, and nausea upon waking. I'm not talking about your typical exhaustion from things like lack of sleep, exerting yourself gardening all day, or having the flu. This is all of that combined and multiplied by ten.

Imagine your body feeling so heavy that it's hard to take a step. You don't want to open your eyes or lift your arm to brush your teeth. The thought of physically having to do anything creates dread. Physical tasks are not the only problem as mental tasks are also taxing. The brain slows down and thoughts get murky. Concentration, focus, and analytical skills are no longer as sharp as they once were. Piercing and throbbing pain causes discomfort and interrupts thoughts. A racing heart, lightheadedness and syncope, sensitivity to temperature, air hunger, and nausea affect your every move. You are trapped on the chess board, and there are no moves left without symptoms.

Checkmate.

Lyme disease, or whichever chronic illness you've been dealt, has you cornered. All of this happened before you even knew you were playing the game.

Since my body operated at only one speed, a snail's pace, it took a few hours to get going. Once I did, I barely possessed enough energy to get through the day. I dragged both my mind and body through this so-called life I was living.

Sitting up, I swung my legs over the side of the bed. I was greeted with aching feet and sore calf muscles. Reaching down with one hand, I rubbed my legs. Shaking my head in confusion, I wondered why my legs would hurt when just waking up. I hadn't been active. That's strange. I reached for a cup of water on my bedside table just as I did every morning. Taking a few sips, I remained seated and waited another minute. This had become my routine. It was important to hydrate before anything else. It also forced me to sit and wait before moving.

It was now time to stand. I slowly slid off the mattress and stood. Walking along the side of the bed and straight toward the bathroom, something went wrong. Within seconds, I fell. Hard.

The fall was so quick and violent that I didn't realize it had happened. Disoriented and confused, I stirred at the foot of my bed. Where was I? How did I get there? My eyes crept open and my vision slowly returned. Trying to call out, I realized I was unable to speak. Completely befuddled and unable to move, I lay there and waited. I could hear John stirring above in bed. He called out to me, but I couldn't respond. Within seconds, he was there kneeling above me.

"Babe? Are you okay?" he asked, placing his hand on my shoulder.

I looked at him and tried to speak. Sounds came out, but they weren't words. My eyes grew wide with fear, and a tear rolled down my cheek.

John could see that I was scared. "It's okay. Everything is all right."

I became aware of pain that hadn't been there before. My head hurt and my lip was sore.

"John?" I asked. I could hear my voice! I was coming to.

"See, you're coming back to me. Take your time now."

I put my hand to my mouth and felt my lip. It was swollen.

"Yes, your lip is bleeding. Does it hurt?"

"Yeah."

I slowly started to sit up, pushing myself up with one arm.

"Whoa, take your time. Slow it down."

Sitting up, I looked at him and saw his worried expression. Reaching up again, I felt the top of my head. Man, was it sore!

"Does your head hurt too?"

"Yeah, it really does. Did I pass out again and hit my head?"

"It seems that way. I was asleep so I didn't see it, but I heard a loud thud and it woke me up."

"This is so strange. Normally my body gives me some sort of warning before passing out. It gave me nothing this time." This incident was far more violent than others had been. It had happened quickly, without warning, and caused injury. I was in shock.

John and I chatted for a minute, and then he helped me up to the bathroom, where I looked in the mirror. Yup, my lip was certainly busted! Great. It looked fantastic. What a nice addition to my work attire for the day. I really needed to get ready for work! I had used an extensive amount of leave and leave without pay (LWOP) and was surprised I still had a job. If I worked anywhere else but the federal government, I would have been fired by now.

"I need to get ready for work."

"No way. You're not going to work. You need to sit and relax the rest of the day."

"I'll be fine. I'm most worried about the way my face looks."

"You need to stay home, Kristin. Are you going to drive after that?"

"I hadn't thought that far but probably."

John stood in the doorway with his arms crossed. He shook his head in disagreement, "We need to monitor you and make sure you're okay."

Ignoring him, I turned on the faucet. Leaning down toward the sink, I splashed my face. The water was cool and refreshing against my skin. I immediately felt a little more awake and revived. Carefully, I patted my face dry with a washcloth. As I looked in the mirror, I ran my tongue along my busted lip, which did look terrible. Grabbing my makeup bag and contact case, I started to get ready.

John wrinkled his forehead and continued to stare at me, not saying a word. I could see his grim expression in his reflection in the mirror. I knew he was concerned, but I didn't have an option.

"Look, I can't sit around here and make sure everything is okay. It is definitely *not* okay, and this is nothing new. You don't have to worry about me. I'll be fine if I just take it easy when I get there. I'll be surrounded by people if I need anything. I can't keep missing work, or I'll lose my job and then how will we pay for all of this?"

John's grim expression quickly changed to anger. Red-faced, he threw up his hands. "I give up! Do what you want; you will anyway."

"John, it's not like that."

"Sure," John said with dismay.

"I have to go to work. I can't keep missing days like this, or there will be no job to go back to."

John continued to look at me but said nothing. He turned his back and walked away with his head in his hand.

I had to go to work. There was no choice. What was I supposed to do?

I finished getting ready, grabbed an English muffin for the road, and climbed into the car. One of my favorite songs started playing on the radio, so I turned it up. Backing out of the driveway, my mind started to wander. Catching a glimpse of my reflection in the mirror, I realized I was unrecognizable. Staring back at me were sunken eyes ringed with dark circles and pasty skin. The busted lip added a nice splash of color to my otherwise lifeless complexion.

Maybe driving *wasn't* the best idea after passing out, especially considering the advice I had received from my doctor the day before. But I could be stubborn and liked being independent. I was determined to push through and fight this illness. Nothing was going to take that fight away from me.

As I drove to work, the events of the morning started to sink in and tears rolled down my cheeks. I replayed John's words in my mind. He had never displayed such anger and disappointment before. John was growing cold and distant, and I couldn't live in denial about that anymore.

Gripping the steering wheel, I monitored my breathing and heart rate. My mind traveled to a dark place, a place that scared me but felt oddly satisfying. It was a place where I could wallow in self-pity when I needed to and sort through my feelings. I was coming to terms with what was happening to me and trying to adjust. I desperately wanted to be well and to feel normal again. I wanted to run and exercise, to smile and feel true joy, to go out and have fun with my husband and friends.

Illness robbed so much from me, and I was slowly losing myself. I could feel her slipping away. Driving would soon be lost too. There's nothing like the freedom of driving a car. It's freeing and exhilarating with windows down, wind in your hair, and music blasting as your car hugs the turns. You can go anywhere you want with roads that lead to infinite places to discover. Going to work that day would be my last chance to drive for some time. Deep inside, I knew that. Another freedom was lost, causing further imprisonment in my own body.

I made it to work and plopped myself down at my desk. I felt horrible but managed to complete a few hours of work and then headed to the break room for lunch. As I stood in front of the microwave warming up my food, my friend Melanie walked in.

"Oh my God! What happened to your face?"

Melanie was about ten years my senior; she was short with brown curly hair and glasses. We had started our government careers together and had been introduced during training. Instantly hitting it off, we became fast friends. Melanie was very intelligent and looked out for me, giving me advice about life whether I asked for it or not. She was a little guarded, but a sweet and amazing friend to those she loved. Being that she was a Type A worrywart, I knew I wasn't getting away from her without an explanation.

"Well… I passed out this morning and hit my head on my dresser and maybe my lip too. I'm not sure," I said with a shrug as I pulled my food out of the microwave.

"What?" said Melanie, her eyes wide.

"I'm fine. You know this isn't the first time." I rolled my eyes and sat down hard at the table.

"Fine? Did you drive here?"

I stirred my food and scooped some up with my fork to take a bite. "Yes, I drove here." As I opened my mouth, I quickly realized it wasn't going to be easy. "Ahh! Jeez, that hurts." My swollen lip was more painful than I anticipated. I put my fork down.

"Oh my gosh, Kristin," Melanie said as she shook her head. "Did you put ice on that?" She sat beside me, her face consumed with concern.

"Yes, I put some ice on it before I left."

"Why would you drive after that? Are you okay?"

I shrugged again.

"I can't believe you drove! I'm getting very worried about you," Melanie said as she leaned in to take a closer look at my busted lip. "My God that looks awful!"

"I saw the doctor yesterday and I'm starting a new medication. It will be okay," I replied.

"Well, what time are you leaving today? I'll walk out with you."

"I leave at 5:30."

"Okay, I'll meet you at your desk," said Melanie.

I had always been a very strong and independent person who didn't want a lot of help or attention. I was brushing her off so I could be left in peace to deal with my emotions about my deteriorating health. I would fill her in later once I came to terms with it all. I knew she was just concerned. I was too.

When I arrived home that night, I called John and we briefly spoke about what happened and how I would get to and from work when I was well enough to go. John was working the night shift an hour away from home and wasn't going to be able to drive me. It was poor timing for us, but it was the situation we were in.

"Call your mother. Maybe she can take you."

"My mom? I really don't want to depend on my mom to drive me to and from work. I don't know if she's available for that. She already takes me to most of my appointments."

"Just call her. I have to get back to work."

"That's it?"

"I have to go. I'm at work. Let's talk about this later."

"Okay."

John hung up.

No goodbye. No I love you. Nothing. I could feel the chill through the phone. The distance was growing.

14

Tiny, Little Pieces

I SAT ALONE SURROUNDED BY the rubble that was my marriage, watching it crumble into a million tiny, little pieces. The wind softly drifted by, sweeping up the bits and carrying them away more and more each day. There they went, dancing in the breeze and coasting into the distance. If I squinted just right, I could see what once was, almost unreachable now. I chased the pieces of our decaying love story but couldn't gather enough to repair it.

This could be the end. The end of our marriage.

As young newlyweds, we were completely ill-equipped to deal with the situation before us. The day we said our vows, we never imagined the "in sickness" portion would arrive so soon. Yet here it was. We were facing it head-on every single day—looking it straight in the eye but completely powerless to overcome it. As disheveled and beaten down versions of the couple who said, "I do," we were unrecognizable to each other and to ourselves.

Staring at my tattered groom, I realized that as the sick one, I never stopped to ask my other half how he was doing. I was barely holding it together myself. When you are in the thick of it, it's hard to pull back and look around. Your loved ones struggle too, and you don't recognize the severity of that when you're the one who's suffering.

One night, we hit our lowest point. John didn't come home.

Since working nights and commuting into the city, John's hours were 3:00 p.m. to midnight; he was usually home by 1:30 a.m. That night, it hit 2:30 a.m. and there was no sign of him.

In a panic, I began to call some of our friends to see if they knew where he might be. Nobody had heard from him. Time passed. By 4 a.m., I was starting to get a little hysterical. My body tensed up and my heart raced. I already wasn't a fan of the night shift commute and not hearing from him; of course, I imagined the worst. Something must have happened to him. Was he okay? I kept making calls. My third call was to Luca. We had remained friends ever since Liz and Luca had introduced me to John.

"Luca, I don't know what to do! John hasn't come home yet and he's not answering his phone. It's late and I don't know where he could be. I'm really starting to freak out here," I said through my tears.

"Okay, take a deep breath. I'm sure he's fine. I'll try to call him and call you back."

"Okay, call me right back!"

"I'll call you in a minute."

I walked out into the living room and sank into the chair. I was always fatigued, and this wasn't helping. I gripped my phone, waiting for it to ring. I jumped when it did.

"Luca? Did he answer?"

"No, nothing. It went straight to voicemail. I'll drive out there and see if I can find him."

"You're going to drive over an hour all the way out there? Are you sure?"

"Yeah, I mean, what else can we do? It's after 4 a.m. Doesn't he normally get home around 1:30?"

"Yeah, he does. I woke up and saw that he wasn't home yet."

"I'll drive out there then. It will be okay. I'll call you once I get there."

"Thanks, Luca," I said, sniffling. After we hung up, I waited by the phone, impatient for any information he might be able to give me. *Oh God, what if he's hurt!? What if he's sick of all this crap and decided not to come back?* I paced the house for a while, wearing a path into the carpet. Eventually too weak to keep standing, I collapsed on the couch. It wasn't safe for me to be alone in my condition anymore. I decided to lie down and watch some TV. A few minutes later, the phone rang. I snatched up the phone and immediately answered it before one ring was even complete. "Luca, did you find him?"

"I found his car. It's still at work, but I can't find him anywhere. I saw his phone in the car, so he doesn't have it on him."

"What the fuck? Where the hell is he?" My worry was now turning to anger.

"I really don't know. Maybe he went out with the guys from work."

"Without calling or letting me know?"

"I can't explain it. All I know is I'm looking at his car right now and his phone is in it, but he isn't. I'm going to head back now. There's nothing else I can do tonight."

"Okay. Thanks for trying."

"Try to get some sleep, Kristin. I'm sure he'll be home in a few hours."

I thanked him, hung up, and lay back down on the couch. I honestly didn't know what to make of this.

Around 8 a.m., I was jolted from sleep by the sound of the front door closing. John was home!

I got off the couch and walked to him as fast as I could (which wasn't very fast), grabbed him, and held him tight. "Where the fuck have you been? I was up most of the night worried sick! What the hell is going on?"

My body was not equipped for this kind of stress. My legs trembled as I stood hunched over from exhaustion. Making my way back over to the sofa, I held onto the wall as I shuffled across the floor. All my energy was depleted. John followed me into the living room, pacing with his head in his hands.

"I was at Jeff's house."

"Jeff? Who is that?"

"A guy from work."

I wasn't familiar with the new people John worked with now that he commuted into the city.

"Well, what were you doing there? Why didn't you call?"

"I'm just tired, Kristin. I needed a break. My phone was dead, so I left it in the car."

"*You're* tired? *You* needed a break? Huh, that's funny!"

"It's exhausting around here! I just wanted to blow off some steam. We were drinking, and I couldn't drive home. I fell asleep on Jeff's couch."

"Who's we?"

"Some people from work."

"This sounds like a bunch of bullshit."

"It's not! It's all about you lately and being sick. We don't have fun anymore. I needed to have some fun."

My thoughts ran a mile a minute: *Is he telling me the truth? What was he really doing at Jeff's? How could he leave me here alone? Why didn't he charge his phone and call at least?*

He had a point though. Fun was not exactly at the forefront of our lives because it had been replaced with my illness. This was all too tiring, and I needed to go back to sleep. I couldn't help that I was sick.

"I'm exhausted from being up all hours of the night. I'm going back to bed, and we can talk more later."

I slowly walked back to our bedroom and collapsed into our soft sheets. My mind began to relax, knowing that John was safe. My body succumbed to the exhaustion, and I fell asleep.

A few hours later, I awoke. Stretching out my legs and torso, I could feel the pain in my joints.

"Good morning, joint pain," I said to myself. My knees and elbows had the worst of it.

I looked over and saw John sleeping beside me. I guess we weren't going to talk about what happened. I hated being on different shifts. We didn't even see each other anymore. I climbed out of bed, showered, and got myself ready for work. My mom was scheduled to pick me up and give me a ride. I told her I was tired and to swing over around noon. I'd work half a day today, which was better than not going in at all.

15

Ships Passing in the Night

FOR A WHILE AFTER THAT, John and I were ships passing in the night. I pushed myself to go to work most days, but we were on different shifts and barely saw each other. I remained upset and hurt by what had happened but wanted to attempt to work through it. We were young, and this was a huge early test of our marriage. I knew we both deserved some grace and that it wasn't time to give up.

Each day I worked, I came home to an empty house and ate dinner alone. The house was so quiet, except for the company of my pets—three cats and a dog. Most nights I ate in front of the television with my dog, Rock, at my feet. Being a 130-pound Rottie/Shepherd mix made it impossible to share the recliner with him. Occasionally he'd look up at me with those big brown eyes to beg for food. I'd pat him on the head and share a few bites. He was always there for me, and he deserved it. We had a strong bond as I had gotten him as a puppy before my marriage. He was my protector.

At night, I would crawl into bed and try to get comfortable. The pain made it impossible, so I wasn't sure why I bothered. After much tossing and turning, I flipped on the TV and watched it until I fell asleep. *Big Brother After Dark* was usually my program of choice. I loved that show. The *After Dark* version went on for a while, and if you fell asleep, you didn't miss much!

John was in the same boat as me. Each afternoon when he woke, he was alone since I was already at work. Financial pressure had grown, forcing me to work more to pay the bills. He had taken the job in the city for the same reason.

I don't know why I was surprised by what happened next—it's difficult to see how dire your situation is when you're the one living in the thick of it. Things aren't always clear when you're living moment-to-moment and just trying to get through the day.

Well, the universe was about to put it in perspective for me. I had an idea of how terrible things were, but life was about to bring me to my knees. My whole world was about to fall apart.

I was sitting at my desk at work when I received a text message from John.

I left a note on the table. I can't do this anymore.

The pace of my heart quickened and my stomach dropped. The room was spinning. I read the text message again.

I left a note on the table. I can't do this anymore.

Anger, sadness, and confusion hit me all at once.

A multitude of thoughts twisted around in my mind like a tornado...

Is he leaving me? What does this mean? Can't do this anymore? A fucking note? Is he leaving me using a note? Is he taking a break? This is not some relationship you can throw away using a note!

I wrote him back.

Are you okay? What are you talking about?

Nauseated, I could no longer focus on his words. My body was entirely too depleted to cope with the stress. Distraught, I stumbled over to the desks of two friends, Eve and Willow.

"Eve! Willow! You have to read this text message." I was nearly shouting as I joined them. "I don't know what to do."

Eve took my phone. "Oh my God, Kristin, what is going on?"

"I don't know. I don't feel good. I'm going to pass..."

I felt myself start to black out and then I hit the floor.

"Kristin, are you okay? Wake up! Kristin!"

I woke up with Eve and Willow standing over me. As I came to, I looked at them, "I passed out again, didn't I?"

"Yes, you did," said Willow. "Here, get up slowly and sit in my chair."

"Relax and drink this," Willow said as she pulled a bottle of water from her refrigerator.

"I can't take this stress, I really can't. I can't take another thing, all of this is too much, guys! My body is literally done. Done."

"I know, Kristin. I'm so sorry," said Eve. "Hold on, he texted you back again."

"What does it say? Just read it to me."

Eve read the text aloud. "It says… 'Forget my note, I threw it away. I don't know what I was thinking. I'm stressed out.'"

"Forget the note? I don't even know what it said! This is unbelievable. Am I just supposed to forget these texts too? I don't know what is happening right now."

While I was angry, I also felt huge relief when the tone of his texts changed to regret and sadness.

"Kristin, it will be okay. You are going to make it through this. I know it has been hard. He is obviously having a really difficult time as well, but he loves you. You love him. You know that. Maybe just go home tonight and talk to him," said Eve.

"Eve is right," said Willow. "You will be okay and y'all will make it through this."

"Thanks, guys. I'm drained. I don't know how much more I have to give." I sat in Willow's chair sipping my water and tried to recover.

"Just go home tonight and rest. Talk to John," Eve encouraged.

"Is your mom picking you up?" asked Willow.

"Yeah, she is. What time is it?"

"About 4:30," said Willow.

"She will actually be here in thirty minutes."

Eve patted my arm fondly. "Sit here with us and we'll walk you out then."

I wasn't looking forward to going home. This would be a rough night.

16

Uncertainty

WHEN I ARRIVED HOME, THE house was empty and quiet except for Rock who greeted me enthusiastically. He pranced over to say hello, his tail wagging furiously. I bent down to pet him, and he planted sloppy, wet kisses all over my face.

"Oh, Rock, you're such a good boy!" I patted him on the head and let him know I had missed him too.

The cats were nowhere to be found. "Missed you guys too!" I called out. It seemed I wasn't getting a greeting from them!

John must have been at work. I made my way into the kitchen, perusing the counters and the table for a note. Nothing. *Phew, what a relief!* Feeling exhausted, I decided against cooking for the night. I made myself a sandwich and changed into pajamas. The couch was calling my name. I sat with my legs curled in, grabbed a soft blanket, and turned on the television.

About an hour later, I heard John's car outside. I sat up surprised. *That's strange. It's not even 7:00 p.m. yet. What is he doing here?*

The door opened and in walked John. Our eyes locked and I was met with an expression of sorrow and defeat that I had never seen before. It felt like my heart had stopped beating. I clutched my chest and watched as he crossed the room to me.

As John spoke, it felt like slow motion. "I went to work, but I couldn't do it tonight. I had to come home and see you."

I felt tears well up in my eyes. "What's going on, John? Are you okay? I'm not sure what to think anymore." Tears started to pour down my face.

John collapsed onto the couch, putting his arms around me. "I'm so sorry," he said.

I held him tight for a few minutes before either of us spoke another word. When we finally let go of our embrace, I grabbed his face and pulled it toward mine for a kiss. His lips were soft and warm, and they felt like home. The faint smell of his cologne lingered in the air and made my heart smile. The passion of the kiss was palpable. I loved this man, and he loved me. We would get through this.

John and I talked for a while that night and finally spent some quality time together. We curled up on the couch and fell asleep in each other's arms with the TV still on. I didn't know what the future held for us, but we had come too far and been through too much to give up. This would not be the end for us.

17

The Absence of Cobwebs

THROUGH OUR CONVERSATION, WE REALIZED, clearly, that it was time for a change. John quit his job so he could work closer to home and return to the day shift. We needed the money that his current job was bringing in, but the toll it was taking on our marriage wasn't worth it. He would be home more now and that's what was important. It was wonderful to eat dinner together again, go to bed together, and tackle little projects around the house when I had the energy.

Evenings were now spent at our cozy kitchen table where we experimented with new recipes, like eggplant parmesan. We painted our basement a deep cranberry red, wrapped the basement poles in creative wood coverings, and set up an area for movies and crafts. We even made our very own brick walkway that led to the front door. When the sun went down and the quiet set in like a blanket over the day, we were in each other's arms.

The boat I felt I had been living on for months on end was finally a little less rocky. The turbulent waters were no longer crashing against the shore; instead, the palpitating pulse of the sea was steady and peaceful. My marriage was on better footing, too, and I was steadier on my feet in more ways than one. The beta blocker Dr. Joy had prescribed for POTS was finally calming my heart to a slow *thump thump*, rather than the drumroll I had grown accustomed to.

What a joy it was to finally have some physical and emotional relief. The storm clouds that had relentlessly remained above my head, pelting me with rain and hail, finally parted. The sun was shining! The sun was *actually* shining! I relished it and bathed in it, feeling it against my skin, warming me to my very core. Feeling happiness deep in my soul and bones, I also remained realistic. I could see the clouds lingering, maintaining partly cloudy skies. But the raging storm had passed for now, and I wasn't going to let its remnants get me down.

John was working close to home, and I was able to get around better thanks to the new medication. Improved mobility is a huge deal for your mental health. Being unable to complete chores for months, such as sweeping the house, is one way to plummet your sense of worth and usefulness. It's funny how excited I was to sweep the kitchen again and how I enjoyed it! I blasted music throughout my home and sang at the top of my lungs as I swept the dirt and cobwebs of my life away. This is when I learned that we take very basic things for granted as human beings. I never imagined the absence of cobwebs would be such a simple pleasure.

Because of Dr. Joy, I began researching Lyme disease and online support groups and forums. So far, he seemed to be correct about POTS, so I wanted to investigate Lyme disease a little further. During my research, I stumbled upon an upcoming POTS presentation by a Professor at the John Hopkins University School of Medicine. It looked intriguing, so I mentioned it to John to get his opinion. He agreed that we should both attend.

18

Postural Orthostatic Tachycardia Syndrome (POTS)

WHEN JOHN AND I ARRIVED at the conference, we found the event had garnered quite an audience. The event hall was large with several rows of chairs which were almost full. I was taken aback at how many people were present. Did everyone at the conference have POTS or know someone with POTS? Not realizing there would be so much interest in a topic like this, I was anxious and excited to see what would be presented.

A man stood at the front of the room beside a large projector screen with a presentation ready to go. This must have been the doctor. Someone was passing out packets of information to each person in attendance. John and I found some empty chairs at the back of the room and sat as the doctor began to speak. He started discussing disorders that cause disturbances in the control of blood pressure and heart rate. He also discussed managing symptoms caused by circulatory problems. I learned so much; it was astonishing to be surrounded by people who understood. I was shocked to discover that there was a POTS clinic in my very own state of Virginia. Additionally, doctors specializing in POTS syndrome can be located in various states and countries across the globe.

The presentation provided me the opportunity to lay eyes on photographs of POTS sufferers for the first time. I was honestly stunned at how I identified with the symptoms and the individuals in the photos. This absolutely was a correct diagnosis for me, and it had taken me a year to get there. I studied the photographs and identified with them so much it brought me to tears—tears of relief.

I had felt isolated for so long. This was validation and recognition of a real physical health issue! One photo in particular stood out to me. It was of a young girl whose hands turned a red-purple color after standing for two minutes, labeled "dependent acrocyanosis."[5] I had the same symptom. Below the photo were doctor's notes regarding patients who had difficulty getting going in the morning and had to lie down after showering. I had had the same symptom for *most of my life* but had brushed it off as inconsequential until it had worsened with time.

The detailed notes in the presentation flowed off the pages like music to my ears. Note after note resonated deeply with me. I became increasingly astounded as the doctor continued to discuss symptoms, all of which I had in varying degrees. "Diminished concentration, lightheadedness, syncope, headache, blurred vision, fatigue, exercise intolerance, dyspnea (labored breathing), chest pain, palpitations, tremulousness, anxiety, nausea, abdominal pain, sore muscles, dizziness and difficulty attending school or work."[6]

When I saw the POTS triggers, my jaw hit the ground so hard I needed help picking it back up. I particularly identified with "prolonged sitting or standing, hypoglycemia, stress, warm environments, prolonged bed rest, hot showers, and sodium depletion"[7]—each of those had been huge triggers for me. The presentation changed my life and saying that it hit close to home is an understatement.

Once it was over, John and I were excited to hang back and chat with others in attendance. We met several interesting folks who wanted to help us. What a community of individuals!

"What did you think of the conference, John?" I asked as we walked to the parking lot.

"It was good. You have a lot of those symptoms. I couldn't believe those pictures!"

---

[5] Peter Rowe, "Update on Orthostatic Intolerance in CFS," (slides, n.p., Baltimore, MD, March 21, 2009).
[6] Ibid.
[7] Ibid.

"I know, right?" I replied with excitement.

"It was interesting. It really puts it in perspective. It helped me realize what's going on." John opened the car door so I could get in.

"I learned a lot too. I feel less alone, and it brought me some comfort."

"Me too." John smiled down at me as he closed the car door.

19

Lyme Disease

AFTER THIS PRESENTATION, I WAS on a mission to further educate myself on Lyme disease, which was thought to be the cause of my POTS. I felt more empowered than ever. It seemed knowledge was key, so I educated myself as much as possible. I read books, watched lectures, and joined support groups and forums. I discovered a Lyme disease symptom checklist created by well-respected Doctor Joseph Burrascano and immediately utilized it for myself.[8] It listed over sixty symptoms, and I checked nearly fifty.

It came to my attention that a few of my coworkers and members of my community were also struggling with Lyme disease and co-infections. Through all my research, I discovered that doctors who specialize in these diseases are referred to as Lyme Literate Doctors or LLMDs. I located a few who were about an hour or two from my house, and I chose one and scheduled an appointment.

Since my neurologist seemed convinced this was the cause of my POTS, I required an appointment with a specialist. I was surprised at how expensive my first visit would be. Members of the forums and support groups had warned me that LLMDs often do not take insurance and that patients must pay out-of-pocket. This is a direct result of the lack of support from the CDC, IDSA, and insurance companies for the Lyme community. The CDC is not in agreement with the treatment or diagnosis methods utilized by LLMDs, and LLMDs do not have the support of the CDC or

---

[8] Joseph Burrascano, *Advanced Topics in Lyme Disease: Diagnostic Hints and Treatment Guidelines for Lyme and Other Tick Born Illnesses*, 15th ed. (International Lyme and Associated Diseases Society, October 2008) 9-10, https://shorturl.at/qyFU9.

insurance companies. Due to a system that is failing patients, the majority of the financial burden of care is shifted and becomes the patient's responsibility. This baffled me and presented a financial concern.

The average individual cost of late-stage Lyme disease per patient was estimated to be $16,199 per a Dr. Zhang study published in 2006.[9] A chart book published by LymeDisease.org adjusted the numbers for inflation and reported that by 2012, the cost would be $20,502 per patient.[10] A more recent Global Lyme Alliance Blog from 2022 discussed how a patient spent $100,000 in three years for treatment.[11] Unfortunately, this is common and families find themselves sometimes spending upwards of $200,000 in a single year. How is this okay? How is it acceptable for a person who is sick to receive no support for their care, or for the care of their family members? The answer is it isn't.

The International Lyme and Associated Diseases Society (ILADS) is an international, non-profit organization that supports patients with Lyme disease and co-infections. They devote their time and energy to the diagnosis and *proper* treatment of Lyme disease.

What's the difference between the IDSA, the CDC, and the ILADS? ILADS isn't intertwined with pharmaceutical companies and corporations who stand to lose a buck if Lyme patients get better.

A week or so after I had spoken with my LLMD's office, John and I nervously walked into my first appointment. We had been through a great deal already and were unsure what this appointment would bring. We sat in the waiting room, looking around at the other patients. I felt already like these were my people, as our journeys had led us to the very same office. As I wondered what they were experiencing, I began filling out the new-patient

[9] Xinzhi Zhang, Martin I. Meltzer, César A. Peña, Annette B. Hopkins, Lane Wroth, and Alan D. Fix, "Economic Impact of Lyme Disease," *Emerging Infectious Diseases 12*, no. 4 (April 2006), DOI: 10.3201/eid1204.050602, https://shorturl.at/eiyCT.

[10] Lorraine Johnson, "Insurance and Lyme Disease: A Problem of Displaced Costs," Lymedisease.org, Accessed October 17, 2023, https://shorturl.at/dLOV8.

[11] Admin, "The True Cost of Lyme Treatment," Global Lyme Alliance, March 9, 2002, https://shorturl.at/bdu46.

paperwork. I was stunned at how thorough and lengthy it was; I had never seen such a comprehensive new patient packet. Just as I was finishing up, I was called back. It was perfect timing, and I was thankful we didn't have to wait too long.

"Good morning, Kristin! How are you today?" asked Doctor Makan.

"Well… I could be better…" I chuckled.

"Aww, I'm sorry to hear that. Tell us what brought you in today."

I went on to explain my symptoms in detail and mentioned my recent experience with a neurologist who had diagnosed me with POTS. He was the doctor who had believed Lyme disease was the cause and had encouraged me to seek out a Lyme specialist. The beta blocker he had prescribed seemed to be working well, and I was able to resume some basic household chores again.

"Do you recall being bitten by a tick or having a rash?" asked Dr. Makan.

Nobody had asked me that before, so I had to think about it for a minute. "Yes. I remember being bitten by a tick in 2005. I was living with my parents before I was married, and I found a small deer tick on my thigh. I don't remember seeing a rash."

"How did you feel after this tick bite? Was the tick attached?"

"Yes, the tick was attached."

I thought back to 2005 and that tick bite. As I began to dredge up old memories, I recalled having strange health issues following the tick bite.

"Actually, I *do* remember feeling bad after that. I experienced numbness in my right leg, unexplained lip swelling, and increased difficulty waking in the morning and taking hot showers. Frequent tardiness to work troubled me. Concerned by the leg numbness, I called the Blue Cross Blue Shield health nurse. As a matter of fact, my dog Rock was diagnosed with Lyme disease that same year. He was barely able to get up off the ground due to problems with his back legs and was treated with antibiotics."

"Is that the only tick bite you remember?"

I thought back to my childhood. I recalled having tick bites when we lived in Pennsylvania.

"No. I did have some tick bites when I lived in Pennsylvania as a young child. We had a large farm behind our house with very tall grass that backed up to our property. My dad would mow paths in the tall grass and my brother and I would run through the maze. We would come out covered in ticks and my dad would pick them off. We didn't think anything of it back then."

"Do you remember having any issues as a child?"

"I do remember a few. I passed out once in third grade. We never did know the cause. Then around age 11, I began feeling *off* sometimes. It was like I needed to eat or lie down. My mom would get me McDonald's fries and that would do the trick."

"Anything else?"

"Ummm… When I was a teenager, I struggled with getting up in the morning. Showers were the absolute worst. I often felt light-headed and had to get out of the shower and lay on the floor. I had a tingling sensation all over my body and felt overheated and sweaty. When it got bad enough, I would yell out for my mother. On one occasion, she fed me goldfish crackers and juice through a crack in the door. We didn't understand or know the cause at the time. My pediatrician diagnosed me with food allergies as a teenager, but he didn't know what foods were causing it. I did seem to react to chocolate, but it was the only food identified."

I was really impressed with the inquisitive and investigative nature of the doctor's questions. I was also impressed with her ability to listen.

"Interesting. Okay, I'd like to examine you now."

The doctor began to push on the joints at my elbows, wrists, knees, etc. It hurt every time she pushed.

"Is it normal for this to hurt?" I asked.

"It shouldn't be hurting you. Does it?" asked Dr. Makan.

"Yes, it hurts every time."

The doctor continued to examine me and asked questions while taking a lot of notes.

"Based on your symptoms and your history, I would say that you've had Lyme disease for a long time. Certainly in 2005 but maybe even as a child as well," she said.

"Seriously?"

"Yes. I'd like to run some tests."

The doctor told me that she wanted to test for Lyme disease and co-infections such as Bartonella, Babesia, Ehrlichia, and others. She explained that a tick can transmit many diseases, not just Lyme disease. The information was a lot to absorb.

As we continued the appointment, we covered my entire health history. I'd never had such a long and comprehensive appointment with any doctor in my entire life. Most of my appointments had focused on acute care. This visit encouraged me to think about the tick bites I had during my lifetime, as well as my health history in general. I was fascinated but nervous and agreed to the testing.

20

Unreliable Testing

A FEW WEEKS LATER, I returned to the office of my LLMD to go over my test results. I sat on the table, looking at the four white walls of the exam room and found myself wondering why the walls were so bright. Why didn't they add some color in there? My breath was shallow and my heart rate was quick. I trembled slightly from exhaustion and worry as Dr. Makan walked in.

"Hi, Kristin, how are you today?"

"I'm doing okay."

"Good, good. I've got your test results here and they appear to be inconclusive. Now, this doesn't necessarily rule out Lyme disease. After examination, a review of your test results, and continuing symptoms, I believe you have Lyme, Babesia, and Bartonella."

My LLMD and neurologist had both now concluded I had Lyme disease as well as co-infections. Dr. Makan explained that the testing available for Lyme disease can be very inaccurate, making an examination of signs and symptoms imperative.

The CDC hadn't admitted to this inaccurate testing yet, but that would change in the future. A doctor cannot ignore the signs and symptoms in front of them simply because of inconclusive and unreliable testing considered acceptable by the CDC. I was grateful that I had found this LLMD. Doctors following CDC guidelines were missing infections, and a growing number of people were becoming sicker and sicker as they were ignored. Pushed aside. Gaslit. Left alone to suffer.

Dr. Makan prescribed a treatment plan involving several antibiotics. These were needed as it's known to be ineffective in treating Lyme and co-infections solely with Doxycycline.

At first, I was hesitant when listening to the suggested treatment plan. It sounded overwhelming as well as difficult. However, I was very sick and everything the doctor was telling me made sense. I had never had a doctor so in tune with the health of my body before. I decided to go for it, follow my gut feeling that it was safe, put my faith in this doctor, and begin treatment with a round of antibiotics.

21

Naive about the Road Ahead

I SAT QUIETLY IN MY favorite armchair, my back sinking into its velvety cushions. I was comforted by a warm fleece blanket and my purring kitten, Smokey, nestled in my lap. I rested there, feeling my joints throb and my body overcome with lassitude. The words the doctor had spoken the day before floated around in my mind like items drifting about in the vacuum of space. As I focused on them, I began piecing together my health history.

I considered the possibility that I may have had Lyme disease as a child and been re-infected again as an adult. There was no way to know if that was true, but I did remember symptoms occurring directly after the tick bite in 2005. I never received treatment for those symptoms and doctors were never able to figure out the cause of them. I realized it was highly likely that I had contracted a tick-borne disease from that bite, which resulted in chronic Lyme disease.

I stared at the long pill box on the table in front of me labeled with the days of the week. Each day overflowed with pills, some small and some so large I didn't know how I would get them down. I wasn't sure what I was more intimidated by—the days with the large pills, the days with the stronger pills, or the totality of *all* the pills in front of me. Suddenly, my thoughts were interrupted when my cell phone rang. It was Liz.

"Hey, honey!" I answered.

"Hey! What are you doing?" asked Liz

"Just sitting here relaxing—looking at my pill box."

"Oh boy, well that doesn't sound like much fun."

"It's not," I laughed.

"Do you want me to come over and make you some dinner tonight?" Liz enjoyed experimenting in the kitchen when she had the time and considered herself a pretty good cook. I loved when she cooked for me. She was the only person who really did except for my mother, mother-in-law, and grandmothers. Her food was also delicious and different from the traditions of my family.

"Sure! I'm not saying no to that offer," I replied.

"Okay, I'll come by around five. Does that work?"

"Absolutely."

"Okay, see you then!" Liz said with enthusiasm.

John walked into the room just as we were hanging up.

"Who was that, babe?"

"Liz. She's going to come cook for us tonight."

"Oh okay, cool. That is nice of her." John joined me and gave me a kiss.

"I'm going back outside to finish mowing. It's hot out there today!" He guzzled down a cold bottle of water, wiped his mouth, and walked back outside.

I felt a little useless, sitting there in the chair while my husband mowed and my best friend offered to cook for me. I also felt thankful and blessed to have support in my life.

I was only at the beginning of my Lyme disease treatment journey, and I was naïve yet about what that meant and what I was about to experience and endure. I had a long, difficult road ahead of me. Things would get significantly worse before they got better; I would soon learn that this is typical when treating Lyme disease and co-infections, but in that moment, I was simply grateful.

22

Felt Almost Normal

THAT NIGHT, LIZ COOKED UP a storm in my kitchen and it smelled remarkable! She wouldn't tell me what she was making as she wanted to surprise me. I typically disliked surprises, but I welcomed this one!

I hadn't moved from my armchair most of the day. I remained cuddled with Smokey and talked to Liz while she prepared the food. We lived in a small quaint home in West Virginia. The kitchen and living room were combined as one open space with vaulted ceilings. I loved how the ceiling opened up the room and made it feel larger than it was.

John remained outside, planting new plants he had purchased for me. Since most of my time was spent at home, he was attempting to make the backyard a place where I could unwind and relax. My only adventures these days were trips to work and to doctors' appointments.

"It smells so good, Liz!" I beamed as I looked at her with excitement.

"No peeking!" Liz replied, a smirk on her face.

"I'm not peeking!"

"It's almost ready. I'll come take a seat with you while I wait." Liz sat in the chair beside me. "How are you feeling?"

"Not great, but I'm hanging in there for now," I replied.

"How's work? I know it's difficult for you to go."

"It's really challenging to get myself in there. Honestly, if I had any other job, I probably would have lost it by now. I'm using the Family Medical Leave Act and that's really helping."

"Well, that's something! I'm glad you have that."

"Are you still seeing that guy you told me about?" I asked.

"Liam? Yeah, oh his smile! I just can't resist it. Liz and Liam. Sounds perfect, right?"

Liz went on about her new boyfriend which gave me something to focus on besides my predicament.

"The food is ready!" Liz eventually declared as she hurried back to the kitchen. She began making plates for the three of us and told me to get ready to eat.

"The food is ready!" Liz yelled outside to John.

John came in and washed up for dinner. The three of us sat at our little rectangle table—a yard-sale item that had been painted with green accents—in the kitchen. It was small, but it was cozy and blended nicely with my kitchen apple décor.

"So... what did you make?" I asked

Liz rushed to the table with a smile on her face and a bowl for each of us. "Chicken chipotle bowls!" she announced, grinning with pride.

John reached for a fork. "Wow, these look good."

"This looks delicious!" I exclaimed.

Liz had made fried chicken and placed it in a bowl atop chopped lettuce, veggies, rice, and a spicy lime sauce. It tasted amazing.

"When did you learn to cook like this?" John raised his eyebrows and sported a mischievous grin. "I thought your best dish was macaroni and cheese?"

"Ha-ha! That's when we were kids. I'm a pretty good cook, you know."

"I know. I'm only teasing you. This is pretty damn good."

"I'm glad you like it!" said Liz.

That night, we sat around the table talking and laughing, and life felt almost normal for the first time in a while. I needed nights like these. I cherished my friendship with Liz and knew there was nothing that could ever tear us apart.

23

The Herx

IT DIDN'T TAKE LONG FOR me to experience a Jarisch Herxheimer reaction, also referred to as a Herxheimer, herxing, or a herx. A herx is a temporary increase in Lyme symptoms that occurs when the spirochetes are attacked by antibiotics. Typically, the Lyme bacteria are "killed off faster than the body can eliminate them."[12] This causes a backup of toxins trapped in the body, which makes the patient feel worse at first.[13]

This is where detoxification comes in as it can assist in relieving the symptoms associated with a herx. There are a variety of methods for detoxing the body, and it's important to discuss the options with your LLMD. Methods chosen, timing of use, frequency, and dosage are all critical and depend on the individual patient and their level of sensitivity and combination of infections.

There are simple tools one can use such as dry brushing, Epsom salt baths, Alka Seltzer Gold, and lemon water. Self-care methods like lymphatic drainage massages and infrared saunas can also be effective at ridding the body of toxins. Then there are binders such as chlorella, bentonite clay, activated charcoal, citrus pectin, fulvic and humic acid, zeolite, and more. Prescription medications like Cholestyramine and Welchol have proven to be beneficial. A variety of supplements and herbs such as N-acetylcysteine (NAC), alpha-lipoic-acid (ALA), resveratrol or

---

[12] Jennifer Crystal, "Dear Lyme Warrior… Help! Herxheimer Reactions, Fatigue, and Healing Without the Use of Antibiotics," November 1, 2022, Global Lyme Alliance, https://rb.gy/h2lsys.

[13] Project Lyme, "Herxheimer Reaction Associated with Treatment," September 13, 2022, Project Lyme, https://rb.gy/bovb4t.

Japanese knotweed, glutathione, Burbur Pinella, COGNEASE and COGNEASE Detox, TOX-EASE, vitamin c, milk thistle, dandelion, slippery elm, cat's claw, Chinese skullcap, licorice root, and so much more also have proven highly beneficial.[14]

I was warned that I might experience a herx, but I didn't truly appreciate the meaning of the word until I felt it.

A herx felt comparable to being on the most terrifying amusement park ride of your life that has no attendant. Since there's no attendant, you don't know when the ride will stop or how long it will last. The ride whips and slams you around, shakes you to your core, takes you through dark caves, drags you through deep water, and then spits you out soaking wet, exhausted and afraid. You think the ride is over, but you realize you have only arrived at a piece of straight track. There are plenty of curves and dark caves up ahead.

Further and further into treatment, my symptoms became unbearable. Plagued with night sweats, chills, hot flashes, daily nausea, dizziness, Raynaud's (restricted blood flow to fingers and toes), headaches, anxiety, swollen lymph nodes, large rashes, pain in my feet and calves, fevers, nightmares, night terrors, poor appetite, air hunger, hip pain, and even sleepwalking, my body crumbled!

Completely intolerant to heat, I frequently visualized jumping into a pile of snow naked to feel some relief. Every day my body felt warm internally, like it was cooking from the inside out. I experienced night terrors so real I feared sleep. Night after night I dreamed of being trapped in darkness, surrounded by nothing but walls crawling with black spiders. The spiders would grow larger and larger and get closer and closer until I could feel them on my skin. I could hear and feel nothing else, except spiders. The scratching sound of their legs on the walls, and on my skin, eventually woke me. As I startled from sleep, my arms would wave and reach to knock off the spiders. My body's attempts to transition from a dream state to reality became more and more violent.

One night, I dreamed of a terrifying stormy sky, dark clouds hanging everywhere I turned. Emerging from darkness, a woman

---

14 COGNEASE, COGNEASE Detox, and TOX-EASE are all products of Beyond Balance.

in a charcoal-colored cloak spoke to me in a raspy voice. The cloak fell from her head, and a hideous face appeared. She lunged at me with such violence that it startled my body into a state somewhere between dreamland and consciousness. My physical body lunged forward with both hands out as if to strangle someone. A blood-curdling scream filled the air and startled my body into full consciousness. My eyes opened.

Immediately, I observed my arms outstretched in front of me, reaching across the bed. I pulled my arms back toward my body.

My eyes shifted downward, and I saw John kneeling beside the bed clutching his chest.

Oh my God. What have I done?

"John!"

He didn't respond.

"John!"

"What? Now you're trying to kill me?"

Disoriented and confused, I tried to wrap my brain around what had just happened. "What do you mean? I was having some sort of nightmare."

"You lunged at me, Kristin!"

"I... What? Are you okay?"

"No, I think I had a damn heart attack! You lunged at me and then there was the scream in the dead of night."

"I did hear you scream. I think that's what woke me up."

"Me? That was *you*!" said John.

"What?"

"Yeah, you lunged at me with both hands and let out the most terrifying scream I've ever heard."

Shocked, I recoiled into myself. I was completely mystified as to how that had happened and knew I needed to put an end to the night terrors.

I looked down at my body and realized something was missing.

"Why am I naked?

John didn't respond, still recovering from what had just happened.

"John, why am I naked?"

"I don't know. That's what you're worried about right now? Maybe you got hot last night." John stood from the floor and sat on the edge of the bed.

I felt my skin and it was wet, along with the sheets which were drenched in sweat.

I took a few sips of water that I kept at my bedside and then walked to the bathroom to pee. With each step, I winced in pain. As I sat on the toilet, I leaned down to rub my ankles and calves and found my pajamas on the floor in a pile.

That's odd. I don't remember getting up, and I don't remember taking off my pajamas.

That's when it dawned on me. I had done it in my sleep! Just as I had lunged in my sleep, I had walked to the bathroom and took off my pajamas! "John, they're in here!"

"What's in there?"

"My pajamas. I must have been sleepwalking."

As I exited the bathroom, I saw John sitting on the side of the bed, still in disbelief and recovering. I slowly climbed back into bed and reached over and put my hand on his chest to try to soothe the stress.

"I'm sorry, John. I don't know what happened. Are you going to be okay?"

"Yeah, it just scared the shit out of me. I'll be fine. I think I'm up for the day now."

"Me too."

During this time, the mental anguish I suffered became so unbearable that I thought I would surely die. I never considered that my body would be capable of surviving this level of pain, discomfort, and complete and total weakness. I ate meals when I could, but only to stay alive. I fought against nausea with each bite of food, and each meal led to frequent trips to the bathroom. Pounding migraines that caused sensitivity to light and odors made me retreat to my bedroom time and time again. Tears welled in my eyes with every step as lightning strikes of pain shot up my feet to my thighs. Waves of imbalance and joints that throbbed overwhelmed me as I tried to move through life. I constantly adjusted my position to ward off pain, despite knowing it never made a difference. There was no escaping this, not even in sleep.

The only hope I had was that detoxing might prove to be helpful in relieving symptoms. My LLMD had strongly encouraged detoxing, so I made sure to follow her guidance. I was happy to work on ridding my body of these harmful toxins. Warm Epson salt baths soothed my joints and, if nothing more, brought me hope. Burbur, a powerful herbal drop, was my favorite as it felt the most effective at ridding my body of the toxins. I also utilized Chlorella, and probiotics and drank Kefir to protect my gut and give it a fighting chance. Kefir (kuh-feer), a thick fermented milk product, tasted like sour yogurt and made me gag every time I drank it. I held my nose and downed it, hoping it would do some sort of good.

Despite the increased intensity of my symptoms, I managed to make my way to work infrequently. I was showing my face as if to say, "Remember me? I do work here!" Part-time work to pay the bills was better than no work. I had no choice but to show up if I wanted to afford my medical bills and maintain my insurance.

I may have been dragging myself in, but every day was misery. While a welcomed distraction, it was incredibly difficult to get myself there. I was dependent upon others for transportation and walking to my desk felt like a painful trek through glass and fire. It was the hardest time in my life. I wasn't sure how I would continue; I was barely hanging on.

24

Praying for a Miracle

I EMBARKED ON THE TREK to my desk, trudging through what felt like thick heavy mud, a hot desert, and knives stabbing into my joints while beads of sweat glistened on my forehead.

The minute I arrived at my desk, it looked like an oasis of crystal-clear comforting water. Finally, a resting place! I dropped my things at my cubicle and turned to Melanie for support. Crouching by her desk chair, I began to cry.

"I don't know if I can keep doing this, Melanie."

Melanie turned in her chair and looked down at me.

"Why? What's going on?"

"I'm completely and utterly exhausted. I feel like I'm barely hanging on."

Tears welled up in Melanie's eyes. I don't think she could find the right words. Other than what she had witnessed of my experience, she didn't know much about Lyme disease. I could see in her eyes that she felt empathy for me and wanted to help. There wasn't much she could do except continue to be there for me as a true friend.

"I'm so sorry, Kristin. Here, pull your chair over and sit with me for a while. You can help me with this case." We both knew I wouldn't truly help with the case; I sat alongside her as she tried to provide comfort while I attempted to calm down. Taking deep breaths and envisioning better days ahead was my only saving grace. It was a bad day for me, and I was lucky to have great friends at work who I could talk to and count on. Work isn't the same without good coworkers, and they truly make a job worth going to.

Somehow, I made it through several more hours of the day and took a walk to the break room to get some water. I was restricted to water as my only beverage, and I was careful to drink enough to stay hydrated. Lack of proper hydration would guarantee heart palpitations and episodes of syncope.

As I slowly and begrudgingly walked down the hall, I ran into one of my colleagues, Jake. Jake was of average height and in his, mid-fifties. He reminded me of a clean-cut, business Santa with his round belly, grizzled hair, jolly personality, and friendly smile. He was never anything but kind to me, and we would always take the time to talk when we crossed paths. When we spoke, he inquired how I was and whether I needed anything. It surprised me how many people had noticed how sick I was and the outpouring of support I received.

Jake was not the only one. Due to being completely out of sick and annual leave, I applied to the Voluntary Leave Transfer Program (VLTP), which allowed others to donate their leave to those suffering from chronic illness or a medical emergency. When several donations poured in, I was shocked. Some donations were from people I didn't even know that well. It was unexpected but deeply appreciated.

"Hi there, Kristin!" greeted Jake. "I haven't seen you around much lately."

"I've been having a tough time."

"I know. I've been thinking about you and hoping you're doing all right. My wife had Lyme disease many years ago and it was hard. I can understand some of what you're going through."

"Really? I had no idea."

"Yes. It was a trying time for us. I know it must be a difficult time for you too. If you don't mind me saying, I've noticed you've lost a lot of weight. You're like a pencil! I hope you get to feeling better soon. You've always been such a cheerful and kind person who continuously has a smile on her face. I'd like to see you smiling around here again!"

"Aww, well thanks, Jake. I know I haven't found much to smile about these days."

"I can see that," Jake replied with a frown. "I want to see you well again."

Jake would never know how deeply his words impacted me that day. His comments were sad to hear but kind at the same time. I had had a cheerful spirit. I was normally always smiling and laughing. One of my favorite things in the world was to help others, serve as an advocate, and bring people's spirits up in any way I could. He was right. All of that had gone away. I had wasted away into a pile of nothing. I was thin, sickly, and sad. At that moment, I prayed for a miracle. I truly hoped I was on the right path, the path to wellness, so that I could find my happiness and energy again.

25

Life as a Lymie

LYME DISEASE CONSUMES YOU. IT consumes your mind, your body, and your soul. Over time, it can devour every part of you until almost nothing is left. You may be unrecognizable to your friends, and many will leave your side. You can even become unrecognizable to yourself. It's an unfortunate truth for every Lymie and for many others with various chronic illnesses. As my journey progressed, I became what we call a true "Lymie."

This is a term of camaraderie for those suffering from Lyme disease. A Lymie is someone who has been in the trenches of treatment or is managing their illness. These folks "get it" like no one else can. We can share jokes about our brain fog, our pain, and our experiences within the medical community. Most Lymies have seen multiple doctors over several years before ever receiving a diagnosis. We, as Lymies, have been through hell and back. We've lost family, friends, our sanity, the money in our bank account, and maybe even our jobs or independence. We have lost faith in the medical community and have become our own advocates. We are fighters. We are warriors. We are desperately looking for light at the end of the tunnel. Some days we think we see it. Other days all we see is darkness.

We are looking for someone, anyone, to pull us out of that darkness. Many days, nobody comes. This is the painful reality. It goes on for months, years, and decades. Our life is nothing but loneliness, sickness, and sadness. Laughter and fun become less frequent and pain more plentiful.

Not everyone is a fan of the term "Lymie" because they do not want to be defined by this one thing in their life. However, for me and many others, that one thing does become your life. It's important not to let it, but so hard not to, especially when you're going through the worst of it. I didn't mind the term because it's what I was, and what I still am. A Lyme warrior. I wear it proudly.

26

The Word Friend

THE WORD "FRIEND" BEGAN TO take on a new meaning to me. What are the qualities of a good friend, a true friend? Do we have expectations of our friends? Do friends say the right thing when you're going through a tough time? Some of my friends did. They said the right things and did the right things. Occasionally, I would receive kind notes, calls checking in, or perhaps even a visit with food or flowers. At work, some coworkers provided support.

Then there were the "friends" who surprised me by casting a negative light on themselves. They weren't there for me, said the wrong things, or abandoned me altogether. If this has happened to you, you can relate to the deep pain this causes. You might feel the pain all over again as you read this.

When sickness consumes you, one thing you discover very quickly is who your true friends are, especially when you're young. At a young age, you live a very active and free life with nights out, parties, and socializing. You get dressed up and go out to dinner, the movies, or local events. Expectations are high. Life is busy. Friends are plentiful. Life is mostly naive and fun. It is the time to live it up, make stupid mistakes, and learn and discover the most you can about yourself.

When I became sick, most of my friends were young and healthy, not yet married, and without children. They couldn't sympathize or truly understand my situation as they had never experienced anything similar. One of my closest friends even disregarded my symptoms completely and expressed they felt it must be related to stress. A few others became angry or upset with me when I canceled plans. I even had friends who made things completely about them. If I missed an event, *I* was the bad friend.

It was extremely challenging for me to go out and have fun. I was sick and I couldn't participate in the activities that I had done previously. I'm sure it was hard for my friends to come to terms with, but many were just not there for me. They were selfish and demonstrated little empathy, not making an effort to meet me where I was or do any activities that accommodated me. The result was losing friends. Some I stopped calling because I no longer had the energy to deal with their emotions and anger. Others stopped calling me since I regularly turned down their invitations. Some distanced themselves because they didn't know how to help or what to do, and they were consumed with their own lives and problems. They stopped calling and stopped showing up.

The friends who remained were the ones inquiring about my health, bringing food, sending flowers, and offering to help us around the house. Even simply sending kind text messages to offer support was appreciated. This is when I learned what a true friend is and what true compassion means.

These were the types of people I wanted to surround myself with—honest, true, real, compassionate individuals. People who remain true friends even when it may not be convenient or as fun as it was previously, and even when I couldn't meet their expectations or be there for them in the way I used to. I didn't expect anyone to drop their lives for me, but it was nice when someone cared enough to check-in.

27

Not a Good Fit

THERE'S NOTHING LIKE CONVERSING WITH a like-minded, fellow Lymie. They provide comfort and understanding and can sympathize with your situation. I developed relationships and true friendships within the Lyme community that I will always cherish. Our paths crossed at work, support groups, Lyme events, and online forums. We laughed and cried together, compared symptoms, and shared information. Many of the more educated and experienced individuals became valuable resources for me. I learned about detoxification tricks, the best doctors to see, and Lyme events such as virtual walks to raise money for the cause.

When I was first diagnosed, the seriousness of Lyme disease was not as well-known as it's slowly becoming today. It was a smaller underground community with scarce resources. We only had each other. Although I found it difficult to attend in-person support groups or events due to my lack of energy and symptoms, I considered it might do me some good to attend at least one. This would allow me to have some additional in-person contact with individuals in my situation.

I learned of a Lyme support group a little over an hour from me in Northern Virginia which was run by a young female close to my age. Since many LLMDs were near the meeting location, perhaps I would meet some people who utilized those doctors and could gain insight and information. It could be beneficial for me and John as I knew he was struggling too. I mustered up the energy and decided to attend.

John and I headed toward Northern Virginia to give the meeting a shot. Since I no longer drove, John took us. We walked outside together, and he boosted me up into his truck. As I stepped into the passenger side, I was enveloped by the comforting smell of it. The gentle scent of his sweet cologne felt like home. I always felt safe in his truck with this strong man I was lucky to call my husband. John had even put my initials in yellow on the passenger side door, to give me a place to call my own. That small, sweet gesture meant the world to me. I sank into the cloth seat and leaned it back slightly for comfort.

As we traveled down winding roads, I enjoyed the scenery of passing farmland. I always felt drawn to rolling hills, old barns, meandering wooden fences, and country homes with large front porches. I imagined a wooden swing in the perfect tree, surrounded by open land and fields of green. What a peaceful existence that would be. The sound of wind chimes in the gentle breeze, birds chirping in the trees, and the laughter of children splashing in a nearby stream, adventure awaiting in nature's playground. Paths among the trees would beckon exploration. I imagined hearing the rumble of an ATV engine and feeling its vibration under my feet. Weaving around the trees, I would pull the clutch and shift up with my foot, accelerating faster. My hair would blow in the wind, and a big smile would appear on my face. That would be freedom. That would be peace. That would be an adventure.

As we grew closer to the city, the scenery changed to busy streets where erratic driving and a lack of parking spaces frustrated us. We eventually found an open space at the coffee shop where the meeting was located.

As we stepped inside, we were pleasantly surprised to find it a charming, quaint little place. It had sandwiches and snacks, and the coffee smelled incredible. I loved the smell of coffee and the way its soothing aroma would travel through a room. Unfortunately, my stomach could no longer tolerate coffee; I sure did miss it.

We approached a hostess and asked her to point out the location of the support group meeting. She motioned toward two long booths where we saw a group of people sitting. We made our way over.

"Hello, everyone. Is this the Lyme meeting?" I asked.

A young girl with flowing golden hair looked up at me and smiled. She appeared to be around twenty-five years old with a lean build and tall stature.

She must have been the leader of the group. "Yes, it is! Join us!" She seemed awfully bubbly and put together for someone with Lyme disease, but I tried not to assume anything. Chronic illness can be invisible.

John and I sat and everyone began to introduce themselves.

"Hi, I'm Emily," said another young girl wearing a blue ball cap. Her voice was soft and timid. She had long auburn hair and looked no more than eighteen. There was a young man with her. "This is Josh, my boyfriend." He appeared unkempt with a scruffy beard and wrinkled shirt.

"Nice to meet you," I said.

"Hi, I'm Alex," greeted a man with thick dark hair and a beard as dark as night. He wore wire-rimmed glasses that didn't fit him quite right and seemed hesitant to speak. His strong square jaw, dark stormy eyes, and sullen expression cast an air of gloominess amongst the group. He was probably in his mid-twenties but outwardly appeared older.

"Nice to meet all of you. I'm Kristin and this is my husband, John."

The meeting proceeded with the group engaging in a deep discussion of emotion, which quickly turned into complaining and wallowing in self-pity over their symptoms. I did not find it informative at all as it appeared to be a place to vent, a kind of group therapy. Immediately, I felt my body tense with stress as I became more uncomfortable. My reaction surprised me. I thought this meeting would be beneficial, but it was only bringing me down. I listened to my body, which clearly told me this wasn't what I needed. Then Emily began speaking about her struggles with Lyme.

"I feel bad for Josh. He is so sweet and tries to take care of me, but I'm sick and I can't do much anymore. I find our relationship struggles sometimes. We are both in high school and I've been absent many days. He misses me when I can't be there."

I found myself agitated as she spoke. How long had they been dating? He missed her when she wasn't at school? These problems seemed insignificant to me. Perhaps it was because I was at a different point in my life and the issues were no longer relatable for us. They appeared to be a very sweet couple, and their problems were very real, but I couldn't take them seriously. I felt guilty for judging them, but I also had to recognize and honor my feelings in the moment. I could tell that listening to them was triggering me instead of helping. Being married for over two years, John and I had struggled deeply and had significant issues due to this illness, issues deeper than this couple could understand at the moment.

Children were not in the picture, and we didn't know if or when they ever would be. Getting better was the priority as my body was no place for a baby, nor could it handle pregnancy or childbirth.

I had to get out of this meeting. It was nearing the end, so I tried to tune the rest of it out and wait patiently in silence. As the meeting finally concluded, we thanked everyone and hightailed it out of there.

A sigh of relief escaped my lips as we entered the parking lot.

"Oh my God, John, that was awful! Not helpful at all! I feel worse. What about you?"

"That was intense and kind of depressing. Much of the time was spent complaining about symptoms. I thought the purpose was to help each other?"

"I thought so too! I couldn't wait to get out of there. I felt myself looking for an escape route, especially toward the end. I just can't sit there and wallow in the sadness of it all right now. I want solutions and positivity. What should we do now?"

John grabbed my hand and smiled, "How about the mall? Do you want to go shopping? We could grab some food there too. It might bring your spirits up."

"That sounds nice!" John knew I loved a little retail therapy when feeling down.

After lunch at the food court, we walked around the mall for a bit. I bought a new shirt or two, and John wandered into Dick's Sporting Goods. It was nice to walk around and be together as an outing like this was extremely rare. After a while, I felt my energy fading.

Slowly, my legs turned to wobbly jelly. With each step, they also felt heavier and heavier as if I were wearing ankle weights.

As we walked out of Dick's, I turned to John, "I don't think I can walk anymore. Something is wrong with my legs." My skin tingled and hurt, I felt overheated, and I thought I might collapse.

"Okay, it's time to take you home," said John. "You've had a long, stressful day. At least you were able to have some fun." He grabbed my hand and put his arm around me to help me stand.

John was so considerate. I gazed at him at that moment and thought about what a great husband he was. John's eyes lit up as he smiled, and small wrinkle lines formed in the corners. His hand felt warm as he held mine. My hands were often cold thanks to Lyme disease and his warm palm was just the comfort I needed. We were both continuing to struggle with the effects of my ruthless illness, but we needed to work through it together. The day had been a good bonding experience for us as a married couple.

28

The Benefit of Support Groups

ONLINE SUPPORT GROUPS PROVED TO be highly beneficial and supportive. I signed up for a few through Yahoo and via e-mail. This form of communication allowed me to pick and choose what I read and who I spoke with and allowed me to gain assistance, insight, and some healing. Through these groups, I learned of another support group that met in person at a coffee shop in West Virginia. Since it was held much closer to home, I considered giving an in-person meeting another try.

I reached out to the head of the group, and she was quite nice. After some consideration, I decided to attend. I would go with low expectations but remain hopeful. If I didn't like it, I wouldn't go back; it was as simple as that. I obtained the details regarding the next meeting and traveled the following Saturday on a cold December afternoon.

John and I got in the truck and headed toward the coffee shop. We were bundled up in our coats, mittens, and boots and could still see our breath in the cold air. Once the truck finally warmed up, I knew I'd have to remove layers. Temperature was a major trigger for me, and it was difficult to remain comfortable. If I became too cold, I developed Raynaud's in my extremities. If I felt too warm I would become irritable, fatigued, and faint. I could never win.

The drive toward the beautiful mountains of West Virginia was far more relaxing than our prior trip to a large, populated city in Virginia. When we arrived, we passed through a small town decorated for Christmas. Adorned with lights, red bows, bells, and a large Christmas tree, it was a stunning sight to see. Christmas was our favorite time of year, and we adored the decorations and atmosphere that it brought.

We were more than pleased as we neared the meeting's location to find a quaint little coffee shop nestled in the mountains. A local shopping center was across the street full of small gift shops that beckoned to us. The window decorations were festive and ornamented as if they were part of Santa's workshop. A little boy stood out front with his face pressed against the glass in awe. He couldn't take his eyes off the train that made its way around a little village. His mother motioned for him to come to her, but he wouldn't budge. She had to peel him away from the glass. As we turned into the parking lot, my attention shifted back to the coffee shop. It was beautifully decorated as well, and I couldn't wait to go inside. This felt like a small adventure.

As we entered, we were once again greeted by the captivating aroma of coffee and desserts. I took a deep breath and inhaled the smells of so many things I missed eating—coffee, chocolate, muffins, and fresh bread. My diet was severely restricted during this time of healing. Caffeine, gluten, and sugar were strictly prohibited and a yeast-control diet was recommended. All dietary recommendations were plastered on my refrigerator, containing the bold lettering FOODS ALLOWED and NOT ALLOWED. The intricacy of the diet and its rules were sometimes overwhelming.

If I wanted to eat fruit, I had to remember only high-fiber fruits were allowed in small amounts; fruits were only allowed at the end of a meal and never on an empty stomach. Certain types of fruits were permitted (grapefruit, lemons, limes, tomatoes, avocado) while others (oranges, watermelons, bananas, grapes) were not. Pears, apples, strawberries, and cantaloupe could be consumed in small amounts only.

The same rang true for vegetables. Green vegetables and salads were okay, but I was required to limit starchy vegetables such as potatoes. Similarly, I couldn't have rice, beans, or pasta.

Fruit juices of any kind, regular sodas, and any drinks with sweetener, sugar, or syrups were prohibited. If I wanted some type of sweetener, Stevia, honey, and Splenda were permitted, but sugar, fructose or corn syrup, aspartame, and saccharin were not recommended. To replenish the normal beneficial microbes in my gut, plain yogurt and Kefir were recommended daily, or taking acidophilus (a type of probiotic) after meals. Water, seltzer, tea without sugar or caffeine, and vegetable juice were my friends. Mostly, I stuck with water or caffeine-free tea with honey. There wasn't much of anything at the coffee shop that I could consume, and the smell felt like distant memories of a past I often missed.

Dimly lit with a fireplace roaring in the entrance, the atmosphere was soothing. A Christmas tree sat in the corner, and the counter that stretched across most of the coffee shop was decorated with white lights.

We scanned the room looking for the support group. A lady sitting by the window with pamphlets spread out on the table caught my eye. That must be her. Rays of light peeked through the window to illuminate her curly, brown hair.

As we approached the table, I inquired, "Hi, is this the Lyme support group?"

The lady stood and introduced herself, "Yes, it is!"

Her kind eyes were noticeable through her dark-framed glasses. She appeared to be in her mid-forties and possessed a warm and inviting smile. I was immediately drawn to her and put at ease.

"Hi. I'm Sandy and this is Amanda. Please, sit down and join us," she said as she motioned to the empty chairs.

Amanda, sitting quietly beside her, flashed us a brief but timid smile. She appeared to be in her early twenties and boasted long and silky dark-brown hair.

John and I sat and talked with Sandy and Amanda for quite some time. It was very comforting and a breath of fresh air compared to the last meeting we had attended.

We were surprised that these were the only two people in attendance, but Sandy explained that others were very sick and didn't often make it to meetings. I gained far more insight and comfort with Sandy than anyone in the prior support group. We spoke about infrared saunas, cat's claw, dry brushing, Epsom salt baths, antibiotics, doctors, some of the struggles we faced, and a plethora of other topics.

When I left that meeting, I felt relaxed and more informed with pamphlets in hand. It gave me a sense of relief, support, and camaraderie. This was a good support group for me. It was nice to finally connect in person with people who understood.

29

Great Colleagues Make the Job

SUPPORT GROUPS HELPED GET ME through the tough times, but so did my job as it continued to be a great distraction from the hell I lived. As I went through treatment, I made an effort to attend work more often. I truly loved and enjoyed my job and career. It was very busy and full of deadlines. Each day required research and preparation of comprehensive legal documents. It was where I was meant to be, and my education and time spent in the legal field had prepared me for it. It kept my mind busy even though I often struggled to get to work and remain focused while there.

Despite my health struggles, I somehow managed to meet every deadline. I don't know how I did it except that I possessed an incredible amount of discipline, determination, and ambition. I wanted to succeed at my job, I enjoyed it, and I was determined to improve my health so that I could enjoy my marriage and start a family. There was so much to be thankful for and so much to fight for. Continuing to go to work through treatment was not easy, and each day brought its own struggles.

As I sat at my desk one day flipping through a file and taking notes, I wondered, *Why can't I find it? I know it's here somewhere.* I had been looking for a few hours for an important piece of information and wasn't having any luck. I made a few phone calls with no success and then continued my research. As I took notes, I was interrupted by the quick pace of my racing heart.

Thump thump, thump thump, thump thump.

Not this again. Heart issues can be so disruptive and stressful. As my heart rate increased, my vision turned blurry, I felt dizzy, and my entire body grew warm. I had been so focused on the task at hand I likely hadn't drank enough water. It dawned on me I hadn't stopped to take a break either. It was time to lie down and hydrate.

I caught my friend's gaze and pointed under her desk. Laura responded in the reliable way that a true friend does. "Need the pillow and blanket again?"

"Yup," I said.

Laura walked over with the soft pillow and blanket she kept under her desk. I climbed out of my chair, spread the blanket out on the floor to make a soft surface, and lay down with my head on the pillow.

"Want your water?" asked Laura.

"Sure, thanks."

Laura handed me the cup of water from my desk so I could sip it while I rested. She knew the drill.

Kate walked by my desk, returning from the break room. "On the floor again, I see. You okay down there?"

"In my usual spot. Yeah, I'll be fine I hope. Just need some time to stay flat to get this heart rate down. The water should help too."

Tracy peeked over the cubicle wall and peered down at me, "Girl, what are we going to do with you?"

I laughed and shrugged my shoulders. "I just like it down here!"

Tracy chuckled and shook her head. "Feel better. Let me know if you need anything."

Melanie walked over to my desk and grabbed my pill bag. "You forgot to add your electrolytes!" She pulled out a packet of electrolytes, tore it open, poured it into my drink, and shook the thermos vigorously before returning it to me. "Now, don't get up until you start feeling better! Is it your heart again?"

"You know it," I replied.

God, I loved those women. The way they all immediately jumped into action, in a calm, reassuring, and helpful way is exactly why I was able to continue working. I would not have been able to do it without them. Anyone who has ever felt support like this knows exactly what I'm talking about, and anyone who hasn't probably recognizes what a difference it makes.

Leave it to Melanie to look out for me and do some mothering. She had become like an older sister, always watching out for me. All the ladies who surrounded me at work were fantastic. Each one helped me in different ways. While support groups can be helpful, it's also nice to have caring friends and coworkers. They are the people you see daily after all.

Unfortunately, I wouldn't always be surrounded by this type of support at work. I would later discover how precious it was. As word spread about my illness, I encountered more coworkers facing the same health challenges. Through pain and suffering, a few of us developed a friendship and were lucky to have each other. We became a core group of individuals known to be informed about Lyme disease. Coworkers began to seek us out for assistance as they struggled to find answers about their symptoms.

We gathered resources and experiences and shared our findings with the coworkers who sought us out. Some of those coworkers were referred to us by the EAP counselor, who had seen an increase in visitors with Lyme disease symptoms. He inquired whether he could maintain copies of our resources in his office and send individuals our way for further information. We obliged. Many expressed feeling lost and alone. We offered support to anyone facing Lyme disease and let them know we could relate. We were all on this journey together.

As colleagues continued to reach out to us for support, I began feeling joy again through helping others. I had been on this journey for over a year while some were just beginning it. Helping them gave me purpose again. I considered starting a local support group in my town but quickly realized that would be too much for me. I was far too sick and weak to attempt to put something like that together. I wasn't sure I could handle a support group quite yet, so I continued to help colleagues within our work community.

30

Lyme Testing, a Tough Pill to Swallow

My LLMD HAD BEEN TREATING me based on a clinical diagnosis acquired through observation and patient history. This was common among LLMDs due to the inaccurate testing available to doctors and patients. I had been tested multiple times, but all test results were inconclusive or negative. Without a positive test—and even with a positive test—it's easy to doubt your diagnosis and question treatment.

Lyme disease and its co-infections are complex and overwhelming illnesses to wrap your brain around, and limited support and research are being done in this arena. In the beginning, my LLMD presented me with the option of a more detailed Lyme test conducted by a lab called Igenex, a company that had grown in popularity due to its commitment to providing a more accurate test. Unfortunately, patients had to pay out-of-pocket for the expensive test ($1,200 or more) as it was not supported or covered by insurance companies. To this day, the CDC and the IDSA continue to support tests that they know are inaccurate despite companies such as Igenex coming forward with improved solutions.

I initially put off having a test done through Igenex because of the high price tag but eventually decided to move forward with it. The benefit of Igenex is that it tests far more bands (specific proteins of Lyme bacteria) than the traditional Western blot, which is a standard test you can receive from your primary care physician and has marginal accuracy.

The traditional Western blot test only covers three bands (specific proteins) for IgM and ten bands for IgG. It requires five out of ten specific bands to have a positive IgG result and two out of three specific bands for a positive IgM result. IgG antibodies are indicative of a past infection while IgM antibodies suggest a recent infection. The Igenex test includes additional bands and has less restrictive criteria, making it less limiting and more accurate in identifying antibodies on specific surface proteins.

When I received the results, multiple bands came back as either indeterminate (IND) or positive. According to CDC standards, this was technically a negative test result since it didn't meet the organization's band requirements. However, according to the standards set by Igenex, it is considered positive if two or more of the double-starred (highly specific) bands are present.

My IgM results reflected that bands 31, 39, and 83-93 were IND and band 41 was positive (++). The number of plus signs reflects the level of intensity of the positive result and can be expressed in one to four positive signs next to the respective band. My IgG results reflected that band 31 was IND, and bands 41 and 58 were positive (+).

While this test result was also technically negative, the doctor firmly believed that this was strong evidence that I truly had Lyme disease and co-infections, especially given my symptoms. The results were highly suggestive because of the presence of one or more highly specific bands. The presence of any one of these bands can be considered indicative of Lyme disease.

In addition, we tested my CD57 count. CD57 is a "cell-surface marker that's present on a certain subset of natural killer (NK) cells—a type of white blood cell that helps wipe out cells infected with intracellular microbes. A CD57 test measures the levels of these CD57 NK cells in the blood."[15] The term CD stands for cluster designation and is numbered "based on nothing more than the order in which the CD was discovered… A below-normal count

[15] Stephanie Eckelkamp, "Is the CD57 Test a Reliable Marker for Lyme Disease?" RAWLSMD.com, March 8, 2023, https://rb.gy/1wwi1f.

has been associated with chronic Lyme disease though no one is quite sure why."[16]

So, it was not surprising when the results came back to indicate that my CD57 was extremely low.

After reading the test results, my stomach sank. I felt dejected knowing that my body was fighting something so fiercely. I already knew I was sick—that much was obvious—but now there it was in writing in front of me, evidence other than symptoms. The doctor recommended we discuss further intervention to fight the infection.

A few visits later, we continued treatment with the addition of pulse therapy. Pulse therapy is when a patient takes certain combinations of antibiotics for a period of time (on Monday, Wednesday, and Friday, for example) for several weeks before stopping them and starting again. The cycle then repeats. There are various methods of pulse therapy, but the idea is that you take antibiotics for a given time, stop, and then resume. I took antibiotics such as Flagyl to attack the cyst form that existed within my body. When Borrelia bacteria feel threatened, they transform into a cyst form and bury themselves within your body or wear a cloak to evade antibiotics. Some antibiotics, such as Flagyl, are considered cyst busters as they can destroy Borrelia bacteria in cyst form.

The doctor warned me that this regimen was going to be a tough one, especially with the addition of Flagyl. I was taking several pills a day now to treat both Lyme and co-infections. These included: Zithromax, Doxycycline, Rifampin, Artemisinin, Metronidazole, CoQ10, Testosterone cream, Vitamin D, Atenolol, Boluoke, Thermotabs, Acidophilus (probiotic), Mycobutin, Bactrim, and Plaquenil. I was detoxing with items such as Burbur and Chlorella and utilizing Ribose Cardio Energy. I was also continuing to drink Kefir and utilizing Nifedipine ointment for flare-ups of Raynaud's. It was a lot to keep up with. I never expected to have a large overflowing pill box at such a young age, but then again, I'd never expected any of this.

---

[16] Ginger Savely, "Everything You Always Wanted to Know about the CD-57 Test but Were Too Sick to Ask," Hoffman Centre for Integrative and Functional Medicine, Accessed August 25, 2023, https://rb.gy/ls4cfw.

Treatment for Lyme disease and co-infections is far more involved than antibiotics and detoxing. It requires taking care of your physical and mental health in ways you may not have previously. I had to learn what foods feed infection and how true it is that you are what you eat. Healthy, clean eating is imperative to healing.

Nutrition is not the only important factor. Mental health plays a vital role in physical health and healing. Healthy relationships, low stress, and habits such as meditation are critical. As I attacked the Lyme disease and co-infections aggressively, I fueled my body with nutritious foods, clean water, vitamins, and meditative moments.

31

An Isolating, Lonely, Dark Disease

LYME DISEASE IS AN ISOLATING, lonely, and dark disease. It will rip your beautiful life from your arms and out of your reach. It can crush your soul and damage the very best parts of you. It is a disease that will reveal all your strengths and all your weaknesses, as well as those of your family and friends. It rips through your life, causing such despair that you're sure you'll never come out of it, and even if you do, you'll never be the same.

As the disease progressed for me, I began to feel more isolated. I found that those closest to me couldn't relate to my disease, my symptoms, or the turmoil I was experiencing. Friendships had been lost, and more friends were starting to pull away as I heard from them less and less.

My husband was exposed to my struggles daily, endured much, and witnessed my deterioration. Our marriage and friendships went through hell and back. Nobody knew the toll it took on us both. My mother helped where she could and she worried as mothers often do. Despite that, our parents, our siblings, and our best friends didn't understand the struggle. We were the ones forced to live through a journey of chronic and sometimes invisible health issues. Nobody was in the trenches with us. That was our reality.

I kept pushing through treatment, reaching down deep for all the strength I possessed. As it continued, I felt worse. The increased symptoms, in particular air hunger, were almost too much to bear. The song "No Air" by Jordan Sparks, featuring Chris Brown, was popular on the radio then, and I can still vividly remember standing in my bathroom listening to that song, tears running down my face. If I listen to it now, those tears come back every time. Every. Single.

Time. The profound pain and fear come flooding back and return me to that moment. Every day I felt as if I were living without air, struggling to breathe, and fighting to live.

Air hunger was torture, and each time the symptom presented itself, it became more difficult to remain calm. The disease had taken all I had to give. Was I ever going to feel well again? How long was this going to take? Why did this happen to *me*? Why is it so hard for everyone to understand and why is there no true support?

I vowed that if my friends ever went through something akin to the torture I felt, I would be there by their side. Even if I didn't comprehend their situation, I would try my best to. I would not disappoint them the way people had let me down. I vowed I would be there in times of need, when they were feeling down, and when they felt like they had lost all hope.

Kindness, understanding, and compassion are the best gifts you can give to the world. Period. I prayed to God to save me in my time of need. I began to pray every single day. Before Lyme disease, I rarely spoke to God. That quickly changed as I found God within myself.

I began to read inspirational books and watch church services online and on TV. I was too weak to attend church in person—as I saved any energy for work responsibilities. I had been raised Catholic as a child, but as a young adult, I had not been deeply religious. I was so thankful that I found God again through this journey. I never needed him more in my life than during that time. When going through a struggle like this, it is so important to find what gives you strength.

32

Deconditioning Strikes

I SPENT MOST OF MY time in bed and felt best in the confines of my bedroom. I developed a fear of remaining upright due to the frequency at which I passed out. Recurrent dizziness and an inability to function normally made life miserable. The lack of physical activity led to diminished muscle strength and a reduction in self-confidence regarding my body's capabilities.

Deconditioning of the muscles had drastically reduced my ability to remain active, and it again became impossible to complete tasks around the house. I hadn't been warned about the dangers of deconditioning or how devastating it could be to the human body. If I had known the condition could develop and progress so quickly, I would have tried harder to prevent it. Once the diagnosis was identified by my doctor, we chatted at length and I conducted research of my own. I was determined to learn how to recover.

As days passed, the condition worsened. Rebuilding strength and recovering from the damage done was no easy feat. "Regaining strengths and functionality (re-conditioning) can often take twice as long as deconditioning. If it has taken one month to get to this low level of function, it may take two months of hard work to return to their original level. It is often said that for every 10 years of bed rest in [the] hospital, the equivalent of 10 years of muscle [aging] occurs."[17]

Without proper increases in movement, I would continue to go downhill. Not only were my muscles impacted but so were my

---

[17] Amit Arora, "Time to Move: Get Up, Get Dressed, Keep Moving," NHS England, January 24, 2017, https://rb.gy/i1952r.

heart and lungs. "Another significant symptom of deconditioning is shortness of breath or a faster heartbeat with minor physical exertion. This is because the heart is a muscle and like other muscles, gets weaker with inactivity. A weaker heart will struggle to pump the necessary amount of blood and oxygen to our bodies, making us more easily fatigued." [18] I learned that even "mild to moderate or even severe deconditioning can occur at any age. The causes can range from illnesses that cause fatigue and immobility; injuries or surgical procedures that cause pain and immobilization; periods of bed rest such as a lengthy hospitalization or illness."[19]

Considering the cardiovascular difficulties I already faced with POTS and air hunger, it was imperative to start moving if I wanted any chance of healing. Since it takes twice as long to build back muscle strength as it does to lose it, I had a long road ahead. This was something I needed to work on immediately. It was time to move! So, I did. One step at a time.

[18] Allied Services Integrated Health, "Use It or Lose it: Why Deconditioning Matters," December 8, 2021, https://rb.gy/x56j9z.
[19] Ibid.

33

Finding My Way Home

EACH MORNING AS I SWUNG my legs over the side of the bed and drank water before standing, I promised myself I would move. Today would be the day. Every day would be the day. Instead of going back to bed, I walked. I forced myself to walk two laps around the house, even if I had to break it up. My legs were weak and my balance was off, but I did it. I pushed myself to walk a little every single day to improve my health.

My arms were like two limp noodles by my side, so each day I used an exercise band for short periods. There was no shame in starting slow. At first, I could only pull the band one single time but it improved with repetition. I continued to push through my treatment regimen of pulse therapy, detoxing, dietary changes, and gut health improvement and slowly grew stronger.

Little by little, my hard work and determination brought an ameliorated quality of life. Each herx became less severe. For the longest time, I felt lost in a cloud of dense fog. As I continued to improve, the fog began to dissipate. It was the absolute best feeling in the world. My mind was clearer, my body felt stronger, and each day wasn't spent in total torment. It was a long hard road, and feeling somewhat normal again left me in a state of disbelief. Lyme disease had taken so much from me. I had forgotten who I was and what made me feel true joy. As the treatment alleviated symptoms, I began to feel like me again. I was happy that my old life had left the porch light on so I could find my way home.

34

Recovery

AFTER A YEAR AND A half of extensive antibiotic therapy, dietary changes, supplements, detoxing, and working on my gut health, I sat in an exam room at my LLMD's office, anxiously awaiting the doctor's arrival. I was feeling so much better, and I was finally getting my life back. As I nervously fidgeted on the table, the door opened.

"Good morning, Kristin! How are you doing?" said Doctor Wright.

"I'm feeling pretty good!"

"That's wonderful! Let's go over your chart and any symptoms. Tell me what's been going on."

I was getting progressively better with each visit, and this one was the best of all. I proceeded to tell him about my decreased brain fog, increased energy levels, and improved ability to function and complete daily chores. I was able to drive myself to work each day, resume exercise, and enjoy hobbies again—and I was beginning to desperately want children.

"I am so thrilled to hear this. I'm looking at your blood work here and it looks great. I have to say, Kristin, I've never seen a case quite like yours. It makes me happy to say I would consider you a true success story! I'd like to discuss it among other doctors at medical conferences and use it as an example for the Lyme Disease Task Force."

"With the rising numbers of Lyme disease cases in Virginia, Gov. Bob McDonnell and Virginia Secretary William Hazel set up a task force in November 2010 to study and recommend what needs to be done... The task force was to study the areas of diagnosis, treatment, prevention, the impact on children and public education."[20] According to the governor's task force report, "There were five separate hearings devoted to citizens of Virginia who had been impacted by Lyme and other tick-borne illnesses. Over 100 citizens testified at these hearings."[21]

The doctor's words rang in my mind. *Success story.* I hoped he was right and I was more than okay with my story being shared. The Task Force was a true blessing, and it was exciting that individuals were coming together for the cause.

Dr. Wright continued by expressing some concern over pregnancy so soon after treatment. "I think it's a bit premature to think of having children. You are finally feeling better, and I don't want you to push yourself. But if your good health continues for a while, I don't see why you can't have children. We can discuss it more at a later date if you'd like, and I can recommend some doctors who can follow you through your pregnancy as that's not something I do. Currently, I am happy to say I think your treatment is complete! We should schedule a follow-up appointment in a few months and keep our eye on you. Remember to continue to take care of yourself."

I was astonished by my recovery. Most days I wasn't convinced I was better, and it felt like a dream. The fact that my story would be told by my doctor was truly unbelievable. I hoped it would help others.

"Would it be all right if I gave you a hug, Kristin?"

"Of course!"

Dr. Wright had been the finest doctor I had the pleasure of knowing. He, as well as Dr. Makan in that same practice, had been spectacular. They were incredibly in tune with what my body needed, always knew what to say, and truly understood what I had endured. I wanted to cry.

---

[20] Laura Peters, "Battling Lyme Disease with the Force," Loud Times-Mirror, July 12, 2011, https://rb.gy/sx5k2y.
[21] Michael Farris, "The Governor's Task Force on Lyme Disease: Final Report," Commonwealth of Virginia, June 30, 2011, https://www.lymedisease.org/wp-content/uploads/2011/10/Virginia_Task_Force_Final_Final_version_7_8_2011_42670 1780.pdf.

I can say that I never loved a doctor before, but I truly cared for Dr. Wright and Dr. Makan. No doctor had ever cared about me and possessed a desire to help me the way they did. It was unprecedented and unmatched.

Through my tears of joy, I told him how much I respected and cared for him. This was the moment in my life when I decided I would always tell people what they meant to me and how they affected my life. I started with him.

35

Pregnancy After Lyme Disease

THERE WAS ABSOLUTELY NO DOUBT in my mind that I wanted children. I knew there was a risk, but I'd already been through so much with Lyme disease, and it was not about to stop me from living now. Research on the topic of congenital Lyme disease was limited, but I had a plan and an arsenal of top resources at my disposal.

Several months after my recovery, John and I began trying to have children. My body had been through quite an ordeal, so I knew it was going to be tough. However, it was time to move forward. I couldn't live in fear. I wanted to look up, hold my arms wide open, and embrace life and all it had to offer. We were both overjoyed that we could continue our life together as we felt like it had been put on hold for long enough. Our marriage was stronger than ever and of course, we were enjoying this time to be close after all we had endured.

After just a few months of trying, I was late. No sign of my period. *Could I be pregnant?* I was nervous and excited all at once. I didn't know for sure, but the possibility alone was overwhelming. I had purchased two pregnancy tests in preparation, so I decided to take one on my own without John. I didn't want to get his hopes up if we weren't truly pregnant. Also, the anticipation was intense, and I wanted to take the test alone to deal with whatever it revealed.

I went into the bathroom and peed on the stick. Then, I waited.

It had a plus sign and a minus sign. Not knowing what the symbols meant, I nervously fumbled around with the box. *Why did I get these cheap tests? Why didn't I read the instructions first? I should have bought one that just says pregnant or not pregnant!* I found the instructions and began reading—a plus sign and a minus sign meant...

I was pregnant. I was pregnant! I was pregnant! Holy shit, I was pregnant! I sat back on the toilet and began to sob. I cried with such strength that I saw my chest heave in and out. This was it. This was finally it! I was healthy and I was going to be a mom. Life was coming together! Then I thought... *Oh my god... I need to tell John! How should I do it?*

I thought all day about how I would tell him. *Should I surprise him? Should I just come out and tell him?* I decided I would do something creative. This would be a special moment for any couple, but especially for us after what we'd been through.

I went to the store, searching for baby items and ideas. Perusing the shelves, I grabbed a pack of pacifiers. Filled with excitement, I rushed home to get everything together. Sifting through a box of gift bags, I found a long watch-type box that would be perfect! It was just the right size for the pregnancy test along with the pacifier. I gently placed the items in the box, closed it up, and waited for John to come home.

Now what? I need a creative excuse for giving him a present. My mind searched for something, anything. *I've got it! His family's upcoming Christmas gift exchange! That should work.*

About an hour later, John arrived home.

"John! Come back here to the guest room! I'm wrapping a gift for the family gift exchange!"

John walked down the hall in my direction. "Gift exchange? It's November."

"Yeah, I know. I'm just so excited about feeling better and decided to do some shopping."

John looked at me with a small, delighted smile. "Okay, what is it?"

Wide-eyed, I leaned toward him and said, "Well, just open it and see what you think!"

"Okay," he replied as he opened the box.

I was so ecstatic that I thought I would explode! My hands shook, and I wanted to cry, but I held everything in and watched his face. John opened the box. He looked at me with a puzzled expression.

"We're giving them a pregnancy test? Ummmm. I don't get it."

Okay, well, that didn't quite go as planned. I waited a few seconds.

"Keep looking!"

"And a pacifier?" he asked.

"Yes... What do you think that means?"

He continued to look at me with a puzzled expression. *C'mon, John.*

I couldn't hold it in anymore. "I'm pregnant, John!"

"Wait, what?"

"Yes, I'm pregnant! We are going to be parents!"

John stared at me with tears in his eyes and immediately grabbed me and held me tight. "Oh no, wait I don't want to squeeze you too hard."

I laughed. He was already thinking of the baby!

"I'm fine!" I said with a smile.

We held each other for a while and talked about how overjoyed we were. Both of us laughed about my attempt at a surprise. Oh well, I tried!

36

Tattered and Torn

MY BODY WAS IN ROUGH shape and had taken a serious beating from Lyme disease. It was tattered and torn and in need of repair. To build back endurance and strength slowly and properly, I began seeing a personal trainer named Karen. We'd met a few years prior when I took her kickboxing class. After a few months of hard work and persistence, I saw improvement.

Now that I was pregnant, I wondered if I should continue working with a personal trainer. I didn't want to push my body too hard or take any undue risks. After much discussion, I decided to continue. I didn't want to lose the progress I had worked so hard to achieve. Labor is also not an easy thing and takes great effort. I felt I should be prepared and ensure I was in the best shape possible.

Since I loved my training sessions and was happy I could exercise again, it also benefited my mental health. I didn't want to give that up. Karen had even designed a music CD that was set at just the right tempo which helped motivate and pump me up. Exercise creates the best feeling. It has a positive effect on the mind and the body and gets those endorphins flowing!

"Hey, Karen!" I said as I got out of my car. She was waiting for me outside in her garage. I always worked out at her house one on one.

"Hey, Kristin! How are you feeling?"

"I'm doing pretty well."

"Okay, are you ready to get started today?"

Although Karen was twenty years my senior, she was in excellent shape. She had curly, red hair and a positive outlook on life. I loved her workouts as they were just the therapy I needed.

"Yes, let's do this!" I cheered.

Karen turned on the music which had a variety of hip-hop and upbeat artists back-to-back. The first song was "Dirt off Your Shoulder" by Jay-Z. I loved that song. As the music started, we began our routine.

"Start by stepping in place, let's warm up," said Karen.

I began stepping in place to the beat of the music.

"Okay, now, let's move to some jumping jacks and then some squats."

The song changed to "Drop It Like It's Hot" by Snoop Dog. I dropped down for my squats!

"Okay, time for some burpees!"

Burpees were one of my favorites, but they were tiring. I could feel my heart pumping now!

The song changed to "Low" by Flo Rida.

Oh, I loved this song! We were really getting into it now. Karen had me doing squats again to get low.

"Okay, time for crunches!"

The song changed again to "SexyBack" by Justin Timberlake. Every time this song came on, I thought of my friend Malorie. She was obsessed and totally in love with Justin.

I worked my sexy butt off as we finished up our routine, and it felt good.

"Okay, that should do it for today. Let's go in and get you a protein snack," said Karen after our hour-long session.

Karen took me into the kitchen and made me a peanut butter sandwich. She was always so good about that. Keeping me hydrated and fed!

"That was the best, Karen. Thanks!"

"You're welcome!"

"Okay, I'll see you next time," I said as I headed out.

"Okay, see you then. You're doing so great! Let's keep this up," she called.

I got into my car and headed home. I could feel the burn in my legs!

John was cooking chicken on the grill for dinner when I returned home. On the nights I worked out, I got home a little later than usual.

"Hey babe, how was your workout?" he asked.

"It was great!"

As I stared at John, I noticed he appeared a little more tired than usual. "You okay?"

"Yeah, I'm fine, why?"

"You just look a little tired."

"Oh, long day I guess," John said.

"Okay. Want me to make some sides for the chicken?" I asked.

"Sure."

"Let's eat outside on the deck. It's a nice night," I said.

It was a crisp fall night, the kind of night where you can cozy up with a light sweater and listen to the bugs as it gets dark. Thanksgiving and my birthday were just a few days away. We sat on the deck and talked about our day and what I wanted to do for my birthday.

37

Dancing Under the Lights

WHEN MY BIRTHDAY ARRIVED, JOHN and I decided to live it up! We went out to eat, bowled a game, and then went dancing! We hadn't had so much fun in a long time, and we both deserved it. Of course, he kicked my butt in bowling like he always does. I managed to bowl a 110 though, which was amazing for me!

The real fun began when we headed to the club. John didn't enjoy clubs like I did, but we both liked to dance. I always loved that about him, and it's nice when a guy has rhythm.

"Candy Shop" by 50 Cent began playing as soon as we stepped into the club.

"Oh, John, I love this song! Let's get it!"

I pulled John to the dance floor and backed that thing up on my husband. I hadn't been able to have fun like this in so long. He laughed and grabbed my butt and pulled me close.

I stood on my tip toes and whispered in his ear, "You're going to get it tonight."

"Is that right?" he said with a smile.

I didn't think a night like this would ever be possible again, yet there we were. In a club filled with people, dancing under the lights. The heat rose as the night went on, and the floor vibrated from the beat of the music. John, with his arm around me, as I leaned back and outstretched my arms, free as a bird, trusting that he had me, and we had come out the other side of this together. It was magical, freeing, and invigorating. The sort of night that feeds the soul.

38

Trouble Ahead

A FEW DAYS LATER, I noticed John seemed down in the dumps and tired again.

"What's going on?" I asked. "Something is up with you."

Something was wrong. I could tell by the look on his face and his body language.

"Okay, what the hell is going on, John? You need to tell me."

"I haven't wanted to tell you. You're pregnant and it was your birthday. I didn't want to ruin it or stress you out," said John

"What's going on?" I asked impatiently.

John glanced down at the ground and mumbled something inaudible.

"What?"

John stammered, "I lost my job..."

"You lost your job?" I collapsed into the chair behind me, thoughts swirling around in my mind. "How did this happen?"

"You know mechanic's shops. This happens. I don't know," he replied.

"You don't know? When did this happen?" I asked.

"A week ago."

"A week ago? And you're just *now* telling me? Wait, what have you been doing all day?" I inquired.

"I've been looking for another job. And I applied for unemployment," he said.

Holy shit. My thoughts were scattered. I was finally doing better, but we had piles of medical bills to take care of. What were we going to do? I was now pregnant and the only one with a job— a job I had barely hung onto. I was going to have to suck it up and pull it together. I would have to support this family until he found a job.

I glanced back at John. He had turned pale and held his hand to his mouth. His cheeks puffed out as if he were about to vomit. He may have been taking this worse than I was. I took a deep breath to calm my mind.

"I can't believe you didn't tell me, but I get it. We've been through a lot. It will be okay; we will figure it out. We have so far. But you can't keep these things from me. We must be honest with each other," I said.

Boy, I was sure learning what we were made of. Was this another test of our marriage? At that moment, I questioned why I'd gotten pregnant so fast. Maybe we weren't ready to be parents.

39

The First Ultrasound

A FEW DAYS LATER, I went in for my first ultrasound! I pushed the job issue aside and let the excitement of the day take over. John and I had already discussed baby names and had settled on a name for a girl but could not agree on a name for a boy. We were in love with the name that we had chosen, and I was hopeful for a girl.

I knew I wouldn't be able to see much at this ultrasound since I was only about six weeks along. John didn't come with me because he was laser-focused on getting a job and working his tail off to find one.

After some time in the waiting room, my name was called, and I went back to see the doctor.

"Hi, Kristin! How are you feeling?" asked Dr. Webber.

"I'm doing great! I've been working out and my energy levels are up. I haven't been nauseous either."

"That's great to hear. Why don't you lay down and we'll take a look."

I lay on the table and watched the screen as she scanned my stomach.

"Okay, here is the gestation sac within your uterus."

I ogled the screen with excitement. The doctor seemed to be looking around for a while and I began to wonder if that was normal.

"Hmmm…" she said.

"What?" I asked.

"Well, I can't seem to find a heartbeat. You are nearly six weeks though, so it's nothing to be concerned with. We will have you come back in about a week and check again."

I swallowed hard as I became riddled with trepidation. I wanted to believe that everything was okay, but was it? I was so used to things going wrong for me when it came to doctors' offices.

She obviously could read the concern on my face. "It's nothing to be concerned with just yet. We will need to wait and do another ultrasound."

I left the office optimistic but apprehensive. I had never been pregnant so I decided that I would remain positive and go back for my next ultrasound.

40

Simple Act of Kindness

TWO WEEKS LATER, I WAS back at the doctor's office for another ultrasound. John came with me. I lay on the table as the doctor scanned my stomach after applying the cold gel. We waited patiently as she searched for a heartbeat.

I prayed that everything would be normal. John held my hand tightly.

"Hmmm..." said the doctor.

Oh no... There it is again...

"I can't seem to locate the heartbeat; let me take another look," she said.

My stomach dropped. John and I waited in silence.

"Kristin, why don't you go ahead and sit up."

I sat up, knowing no good news was coming.

"I'm so sorry, but I'm not able to find a heartbeat."

"What does that mean?"

"Well, it appears that the baby is not developing."

"What? I don't understand."

"Well, it looks like what we call a blighted ovum. That is when the egg is fertilized and implants into your uterus but fails to develop," she explained.

John and I gazed at each other with sadness in our eyes. Tears streamed down my face.

The doctor touched my shoulder. "I'm so sorry, Kristin and John. I know this is difficult to hear," she said.

I appreciated her genuine concern. Tears welled up in her eyes as well. I couldn't believe this was happening. I just wanted to run out of the room.

"You have a few options. You can wait for a miscarriage to occur, or we can do what's called a D and E."

As the doctor went on to explain the options, my mind trailed off and I became lost in my thoughts. I just wanted to leave.

"I just want to go home. Can I think about it?"

"Of course, you can. Do you want to come back at about nine weeks and we can decide then?"

"That's fine," I said.

John and I left with a great deal of sadness in our hearts. We were still in shock, but beyond that, we felt grief. It was the most profound grief I had ever felt in my life. Just when I thought things were looking up, life had taken another turn.

Days passed with clouds of darkness looming over our heads and in our hearts. I didn't want to talk to anyone, and I didn't want to go anywhere. I decided to take a leave of absence from work so we could focus on deciding. With John still looking for employment, time off made me uneasy, but I knew I couldn't worry about that.

As I wrestled with the decision, I spoke to some friends and family that were aware of my pregnancy. This would become another time in my life when I learned that people don't always react in the ways you'd expect them to. Some friends and family were very sweet, but others said all the wrong things. I suspected this may have been because they had never lost a child before. The loss of a child at any point during a pregnancy results in tremendous grief. It's a pain that can't be explained to others.

One friend chose this time to confide in me about a past trauma she had experienced. I knew she was only trying to relate and comfort me, but it was not helpful nor the appropriate time to share it. Another family member had the audacity to say, "I'm not sure why you're so sad. It was never really a baby." That one stung the most. It was as if they were disregarding my grief completely and were disconnected from the situation.

Why was it that with every difficult situation I faced nobody seemed to understand my pain? The complete and utter sorrow, grief, anguish, torture, and agony that plagued my life with Lyme disease caused me to feel so alone. Now, I was alone again dealing with the profound loss of a child, which no one in my life seemed to understand.

The hardest part was not knowing why it happened. Was my body not ready because of Lyme disease? Was it something I did? Did I exercise too much? Was it something out of my control? There was no way to know.

One simple act of kindness by a friend stood out to me.

It wasn't anything spectacular or expensive, and it wasn't anything that they said. Willow sent me flowers. For some reason, not a single person in my life thought to do this except her. I don't know the appropriate response when a friend has a miscarriage, but I know it showed me she cared.

When the flowers arrived, I smiled and cried. They somehow represented something completely different to me than they would have in the past. I observed those flowers every single day, watching them blossom and grow. It became a reminder to me that life could grow within me once again. This was not the end. This was only the beginning of my pregnancy journey. Everything would be okay.

41

The Decision

THE DECISION I HAD TO make next was an extremely personal one. Nobody should tell you what to do, and only you know what you can emotionally handle and what is going to help you heal. I decided I couldn't have something inside of me that wasn't growing. If no baby was developing, then I needed to move past this as it was emotional torture.

My sister-in-law, Therese, was the only person other than John whom I was able to have a conversation with about this and who openly supported my decision. I was so thankful for my lengthy discussions with her. She completely understood why I needed to do this and helped talk me through it.

The other issue regarded our finances. I absolutely could not afford to miss any additional time from work. I had to go back, and I was nervous I would have a miscarriage while I was there. That is something I didn't want to go through as I had witnessed it happen to someone else.

At approximately ten weeks, I went back to the doctor for a scheduled D and E (dilation and evacuation). I met her at the hospital where I was prepped for the procedure. As I lay in the hospital bed, emotions overcame me. I felt immensely alone and despondent. Before the procedure began, the doctor came in to talk to me. I looked up at her, tears rolling down my face.

"This is awful," I cried. "I've never felt such intense emotional pain."

The doctor grabbed my hand and held it tight. I saw a tear roll down her cheek. As we cried together, it was a strangely therapeutic moment. I could tell she knew how horrible this was for me—removing the life from me that never had a chance.

"Please, just take care of me," I said.

The doctor squeezed my hand again and said she would see me afterward.

After the procedure, I spent most of my time on the sofa, sobbing and writhing in pain. I suffered from severe cramping and was required to monitor anything I passed, such as clots. The grief was unbelievably strong. I wanted to hibernate and be left alone.

I insisted that no one come to visit as I wanted to grieve in peace. Of course, my stubborn and worried father showed up anyway with my mother in tow. He stood over me with downcast eyes and a frown, paralyzed, knowing there was nothing he could do.

A few weeks passed, and I went back to work like nothing had happened. I didn't tell anyone what had occurred. They all assumed I had surgery due to recent back pain. I let them all think it was true. Not many people even knew I had been pregnant. It would have been too hard to face everyone at work—the sad faces, the "I'm so sorry for your loss" statements. I wanted to skip that part. I needed to deal with the grief in my own way and in my own time. My heartache went on for several months. I knew it was something that would never go away, but maybe it could get better. After about five months, John and I discussed whether we wanted to try again.

"What do you think?" I asked.

"I think we should go for it. The doctor said it would be safe to try again once we gave your body a few months to heal. But what do you want?" he asked.

"I want to try again. Maybe it will help us heal. I don't want to sit around being sad and not try. We've been through so much already and now I'm twenty-seven years old. I feel like the clock is ticking."

"Okay, well, then let's do it. As long as you're sure," he said.

"Well, I don't know that I'm sure of anything, but we should try. I want to try," I said.

I scheduled a follow-up appointment with my OB to let them know John and I planned to try again. At the appointment, the doctor said they wanted to do some investigating as to the cause of my miscarriage. I agreed to let them run some tests. I assumed I had tried too soon after Lyme disease and my body wasn't ready. The OB explained that there are many reasons women miscarry and the blood work may be able to find a cause.

42

MTHFR (It's Not What You Think)

I SAT IN AN EXAM room at the OB's office once again. They had called me in to go over the blood work results in person, which is never a good sign. I fidgeted in my chair as I waited for the doctor to come in, unaware that I was about to learn something new and unexpected about myself. Finally, the doctor arrived.

"Kristin, your results are back, and they show you have what's called an M-T-H-F-R mutation."

"What?" I asked.

"It means you have a mutation in the MTHFR gene. This can be hereditary, and it could potentially be what caused your miscarriage. There really is no way to know for sure."

"I've never heard of this before," I said.

"It can put you at an increased risk for complications during pregnancy or can cause miscarriage and other health issues."

At that moment, I just couldn't help it. I started laughing!

I went through actual hell with Lyme disease and now I had discovered that I have a genetic mutation that looks like a curse word! Well, if this isn't a motherfucker!

The doctor looked at me, perplexed.

"I'm just laughing at the irony of all of this. It's either this or cry, and I'm sick of crying."

"I understand. I'm going to give you a prescription for an excellent prenatal vitamin you can take. It should help support your body while you try to conceive again."

I thanked her and left the office. But I couldn't help but feel a little angry. If a gene defect like this can cause miscarriages, why weren't doctors testing women for it? Why were we waiting until women lost their babies before we figured it out? It was preposterous to me. But this was only the first thing I'd discover on a long journey. It was also my introduction to genetics and how they can play a role in our health.

43

Congenital Lyme

ATTEMPTING TO GET PREGNANT AGAIN was an emotional journey. Without knowing the true cause of the miscarriage, it felt like we were playing roulette. We didn't know what the future would hold for us, and we prayed that everything would work out. Shockingly, just a few months later, I became pregnant again. John and I were over the moon. We knew in our hearts everything would be okay this time around. We just knew it. The hope we held in our hearts was healing and positive for us. We dusted the baby name book off the shelf and began looking at names again. Nothing had changed. We still could not decide on a boy's name, but we easily agreed upon a name for a baby girl.

At my first ultrasound appointment, I was terrified. I needed to hear the baby's heartbeat so I would know everything was okay. I felt in my heart and my gut that all would be fine, but I was still scared until I knew for sure.

I found myself, yet again, in one of those flattering paper gowns lying on a table and holding John's hand. I swear I held my breath until I heard it... *Thump, thump... Thump, thump... Thump, thump.*

"John, the heartbeat!" I exclaimed.

"It's so fast," he said.

"That's normal," said the doctor. "It sounds like a strong heartbeat!"

John and I couldn't have been happier in that moment. We looked at each other with so much joy in our eyes and a sense of relief. God, let this be a successful pregnancy and a happy, healthy baby.

When I returned home that night, I opened the pregnancy journal I had kept during my first pregnancy. As I read it, I could feel the excitement and joy I had felt back then flowing from the pages. It was sad to read through my elation as it was clear that the thought of losing the baby had never crossed my mind. I said a prayer and set the journal to the side. I rubbed my belly and spoke to the life growing inside.

"This time will be different, my sweet baby. I'm going to take good care of you, and everything will be all right," I said.

I changed things up for this pregnancy and only engaged in light exercising, refraining from personal training and heavy cardio. I wasn't told this played a role in my miscarriage, but I wasn't about to take any chances. I took the prenatal vitamin my OB suggested every day and continued care under my new LLMD.

Since my prior Lyme doctor did not take on pregnant patients, I had moved to a new doctor he recommended. She was wonderful and compassionate. She once again treated me with antibiotics during my pregnancy and instructed me to continue hydrating with water only and to eat healthily. Many of the same dietary guidelines were still in play, as it would hopefully give my body the best chance at maintaining my good health.

Separately, I also reached out to Dr. Jones, a widely known Lyme pediatrician and pioneer in the treatment of children. His kindness, empathy, and knowledge were evident during our conversations. He informed me what treatment had been successful for pregnant women in his experience and assured me I was on the right track. I'll never forget the impact his reassurance and knowledge had on my pregnancy. He gave me the confidence and hope I needed.

Deciding whether to have children after Lyme is an extremely personal, emotional, and difficult decision. Knowing that I had some of the best doctors on my team put me at ease. A team of qualified, knowledgeable, and compassionate healthcare practitioners is necessary for a pregnant woman with Lyme disease. There is a real risk of congenital Lyme and once we have experienced the horrors of the disease, it is the last thing we would ever wish on our children. Unfortunately, information on congenital Lyme disease is not something pregnant women are provided even though it was discovered over thirty-five years ago. "Though scientists have known Lyme is congenital since 1985, it took the CDC until 2020 to finally acknowledge this fact."[22]

Not only did I have this complication, but my discovery of the MTHFR mutation also made my pregnancy high risk. A high-risk OB, who also happened to be Lyme-friendly and understood the risks, followed me during my pregnancy. With two OBs and two LLMDs on my side, I felt confident I was doing all that I could to protect my baby. I used everything available in my arsenal, and that's all I could do.

Of course, that didn't mean I didn't feel immense pressure on my shoulders and the added concern that came with my situation. This was no ordinary pregnancy, and I felt the gravity of my situation every day. Nobody in my life, not even John, truly understood what it was like to worry about these things while pregnant. In the back of my mind also lived the constant fear of returning symptoms and the potential of the inability to care for my child.

I was very fortunate that, for the most part, my pregnancy went very well. A few months in, I was feeling pretty good. I suffered from nausea, but I really couldn't complain. I didn't throw up once, and other than the typical nausea, there were no other issues of note. I also discovered some positives to pregnancy. My hair became incredibly shiny, soft, and curly. I already had wavy hair, but my hair curled right up in tight, beautiful curls. It had never looked so amazing! My skin began to glow, and the hair on my legs started growing very slowly. Now I could work with *this*!

Feeling life move inside me was incredible. In some respects, it did feel strange. The thought of a human being growing inside of me was both astonishing and mysterious.

John and I decided we wanted to know the gender of the baby. I had a gut feeling that it would be a boy.

As I sat in the waiting room of the OB's office, that gut feeling suddenly changed. An overwhelming feeling washed over me. No, this was a girl. I was sure of it; this was a girl. I knew it in my bones.

---

[22] "Congenital Lyme," March 16, 2021, Project Lyme, https://rb.gy/nne4xg.

I turned out to be correct; it was a girl! We were very happy, especially since we had already agreed on a beautiful name.

My friends and family were thrilled for us, and my two best friends threw us a baby shower. In fact, we had *two* baby showers! Some of my mother-in-law's friends also threw a shower. We received many wonderful and generous gifts. I felt the outpour of love and relief as we didn't have a lot of money for baby items. John had been without a job for a few months and had recently started working somewhere new.

A local mechanic shop had given him a job. It was a blessing, and I was very thankful to them. The hours were fantastic, Monday through Friday 8:00 a.m. to 5:00 p.m., and no weekends! We didn't have a lot of money as we were playing catch up and still paying medical bills. We were thankful for our nice, cozy home and started making a beautiful nursery for our baby girl.

I picked out two colors for the nursery, a soft, calming pink and a cream color. We painted the top half of the walls pink and the bottom cream with a chair rail. I went with a theme I loved from my childhood, Hello Kitty. We visited Babies R Us and bought a few brand-new items on our own. We picked out a light-colored wood crib, a changing table, and a blush pink blanket that read, "Beautiful like mommy."

We also bought a crib mattress and some other small items. We purchased a light-colored wood dresser from a yard sale and lined it with adorable baby wrapping paper. I filled the changing table with diapers and little onesies. I washed the baby clothes we received, folded them, and put them away in the dresser. The nursery looked great—simple, beautiful, and perfect. I placed a glider in the corner. My mother, a gifted quilt-maker, made a gorgeous quilt for the baby. I folded it neatly over the back of the glider. I couldn't wait to rock my baby in this beautiful nursery.

As the pregnancy progressed and my belly grew, I saw baby feet and hands poke out from my stomach. It looked like a little alien trying to escape! What a neat experience. I read stories to my baby girl and even put headphones against my stomach with music playing. Part of me thought maybe the miscarriage had happened for a reason. It certainly made me appreciate every moment of this pregnancy. I recorded everything and enjoyed every moment. I held onto every physical and emotional feeling. I managed to get everything that's recommended in pregnancy books for new moms such as a wipe warmer, a swing, a Bumbo seat, multiple types of bottles, etc. I wanted to have everything in case I needed it. Preparation calmed me.

44

Giving Birth

ON DECEMBER 7, I THOUGHT I felt contractions. It was very early in the morning, and they hit strong. That couldn't be right. It was the baby's due date, Pearl Harbor Day! I had read that it is very rare for a baby to come on its due date. For some reason, a wave of calm came over me and I was at peace. I felt so much joy. I let John sleep as I jumped in the shower. Once I was clean and dressed, I grabbed my bags. The contractions were stronger now and only two minutes apart. This was happening fast.

I gently tapped John on the shoulder. "John, wake up. It's time."

John rolled over and slowly opened his eyes. "What?"

"It's time. I'm having contractions."

"Right now?"

"Yes. Well, they have been happening for about thirty minutes, but I let you sleep."

John quickly sat up and jumped out of bed. "What? You should have woken me up! Let's get the bags."

"I've already got them."

John gawped at me with raised eyebrows, "You do? Wow, are you ready to go?"

"Yeah, pretty much." I was ready to do this!

"Okay, I'll get dressed, and we'll go." John threw on some pants, and we were out the door.

We got in the car and headed to the hospital. Once we arrived, the nurses hooked me up to monitors. Labor progressed quickly. I wasn't there long before the nurses placed me in a room. My mom met us there.

"A room already?" I asked.

"Yes, ma'am. You are six centimeters, hon! Let's go ahead and get you in a gown."

"Six centimeters already?" I was surprised at how easy it was.

As I continued to labor, I asked the nurses if they were aware that I wanted to test the cord blood and placenta for Lyme disease. I had communicated this with my OB and had told the hospital previously and included it in my paperwork. Despite my attempts to communicate the information, the staff was completely unaware. I became frustrated and wondered why nobody discussed this request that had been part of my birth plan for months.

They were missing important documents, so I called my LLMD while in labor. I began calling her office and e-mailing her repeatedly. John helped me. After what felt like forever, John was able to reach her, and she faxed some paperwork over to the hospital. How absurd that I had to do this while in labor! Where was the doctor?

Once it was squared away, I was able to focus more on my labor. I was not having this baby without the cord blood test first being ready to go. As labor progressed, the nurse informed me it was my last chance to get an epidural. The staff really pushed it. I decided to get one mostly out of fear, fear of how intense the labor pain would get.

Once the epidural kicked in, I couldn't feel the lower half of my body. I knew this was the desired effect, but my body did *not* like it and began to feel strange. Something was wrong. I just knew it. I felt sick and had trouble breathing. I laid back in my hospital bed and tried to relax. The machines and monitors in the room beeped and chimed, surrounding me with a distressing symphony of noises. Nurses began flying in, flooding the room with people I didn't know. The air was permeated with fear and concern. One of the nurses placed an oxygen mask over my mouth and nose.

"You and your baby need this oxygen, sweetie. Take several deep breaths, relax, and focus on your breathing," she said.

The baby's heart rate was rising, and I needed to breathe to save her. I knew this was not the time to panic. I was surrounded by nurses and the doctor, and I could hear my mom panicking on one side of the room. Out of the corner of my eye, I saw John dressing in scrubs.

I closed my eyes and blocked everything out of my mind except my breathing. Slowly, the people, the noises, and the fear that filled the room with negative energy began to disappear. I lay there and calmly breathed the oxygen and focused on my baby. It was just me and my baby girl in the room.

I felt someone touch my arm. I opened my eyes, and the doctor had taken a seat beside me.

"I don't want to alarm you, but I need to quickly present you with some options, and we need to act fast."

She explained that the baby was in danger and not getting enough oxygen. She thought we needed to move to an emergency cesarean. I was not prepared for this, and I was scared but I didn't hesitate.

"Do whatever you have to do to protect my baby," I said.

I attempted to think zero negative thoughts and remained present in those moments. The nurses wheeled me into an operating room. Since I had an epidural, they were able to quickly numb me in preparation for surgery. It all happened so fast and before I knew it, the operation had begun.

The experience of the birth of my first child was not at all what I had expected. In fact, most of it was quite terrible. The details of an emergency caesarian had never been explained to me, and I was certainly never told that I could potentially be tied down to a table, completely unaware of what was happening. Even though I was awake, no one was talking to me. I felt like a spectator to some barbaric event in which I was the main character. Even when I spoke, nobody replied except the anesthesiologist who was of no use at all. He didn't answer any of my questions and continuously tried to distract me. I guess this was their strategy for handling pregnant women tied to a table, but it wasn't working. I'm the kind of person who likes to know what is going on and that everything is fine. Details and reassurance are what calm me.

It was not a pleasant or mentally healthy experience. The entire caesarian felt like a violation. I had already been through quite a lot and wanted to protect my baby, yet had absolutely no control over the situation.

When they lifted my baby girl from my body, it was a bizarre feeling and emotionally damaging. One minute your baby is protected inside your body and the next it's ripped from your insides. It did not feel natural. Instead, it felt like complete and total emptiness. It felt like someone had taken my baby from me in one swift movement.

I wondered why women talk about how they prefer cesareans, believing them to be easier and less painful. I wished women were encouraged to trust what their bodies were born to do, and what women have been doing for thousands of years. The doctor came around the curtain, held the baby up to my head, and had the nurse take a few pictures. I stared longingly at her beautiful face. I was shocked at the similarities of our facial features. I could see her father in her eyes and forehead, and I could see myself in her mouth and chin.

In another swift movement, my baby was taken from me again. The nurses and doctor cleaned her up and then rolled me to a recovery room where I waited, and waited, and waited. The room was very small with plain white walls and bright lighting. You couldn't fit much into this square room except my hospital bed. It was claustrophobic and lonely. I kept falling in and out of consciousness from the exhaustion and morphine they had administered. It felt like I was away from my baby for an eternity. I wondered where my husband was, my mom, the nurses, anyone! But most of all, I was left wondering where my baby was and whether she was okay.

Eventually, I was moved from the recovery room to an actual room. The minute they brought my baby girl to me, I demanded to hold her skin-to-skin! I vowed at that moment that I would never have another cesarean or epidural again if I could help it.

The next day, exhaustion and emotion began to take over my mind and body, and the nurses identified that I possessed the signs of baby blues.

They closed off my room to visitors and insisted I rest as much as possible for twenty-four hours. As I attempted to rest and bond with my baby, family members called and texted John over and over. They were upset that they were not able to see the baby and were giving him a hard time. The selfish display of family members, as I lay there suffering and recovering, was deeply upsetting. After all John and I had been through, this is how they chose to behave, putting pressure on John and making things about them.

Weeks later, once we were home and settled with our new baby girl, we received the cord blood test results. The result was *positive* for Lyme bacteria. It was considered the first documented case of Lyme disease transmitted from mother to fetus in our state. Despite being treated for Lyme throughout my pregnancy, the bacteria had made its way into the cord blood. The news was devastating and utterly soul-crushing. I felt I had endangered my child. The treatment was not successful. Why hadn't it worked? The only thing I could do was continue treatment while breastfeeding. Maybe my breast milk would make my baby stronger?

As every mother knows, deciding whether to breastfeed is a hugely personal decision, and in my situation, there was an added risk. Despite this added risk, there was almost no guidance for women in my position. We located an LLMD that was willing to see and treat newborns and children and scheduled a physical. The thorough exam was both nerve-wracking as well as comforting. I felt my baby was in capable hands and that they were doing everything they could with what information we had to date.

The exam involved another Lyme disease test as we were to test her both at infancy and at age one. At our second visit, we were provided with the results of the test, which showed an unbelievably powerful antibody response to Lyme. It was very upsetting to see her body working so hard to fight this bacterium that I had exposed her to. Due to the test results, as well as the presentation of acid reflux, she was prescribed antibiotics to mix in a bottle with her formula. By the time this medication was prescribed, I was having difficulty with breastfeeding and supplementing with formula. This made administering the medication fairly easy. Despite the prescription of medication, the results of the exam were that we had a happy, healthy baby. We were advised to test her again at age one and to continue to observe her for any symptoms.

45

Vaginal Birth After Cesarean (VBAC)

JOHN AND I WERE BLESSED to get pregnant a third time less than one year later. I hired a doula and created a birth plan as I was determined to make this birth a positive experience.

I would stay home as long as possible during labor with no intervention by medical staff unless there was an emergency and no pain medication. The goal, and my desire as a mother, was to achieve the most natural and organic birth possible.

Since the birth of our first daughter, I suffered from dreadful pain in my spine around the site of the epidural injection. Touching the area caused great discomfort, including wearing a bra. This was another reason I was adamantly against a second epidural.

It was not easy to find a doctor who would support a VBAC (vaginal birth after cesarean). For some reason, many doctors in my area feared a VBAC and tried to frighten and intimidate me into changing my mind. The doctor who had delivered my first baby insisted that if an emergency occurred, she could be forced to cut me open on a table without pain medication. She feared that without an epidural needle being placed, they would have no way to quickly deliver medication. Determined to arm myself with information and not act out of fear again, I conducted research and spoke to doctors outside my area and to my doula. I even took birthing classes. I requested copies of my medical records to join a different practice, but the office administrator told me that if I left, I'd never be allowed back. I hadn't yet been able to find a replacement with an opening, so I felt stuck. Threats seemed to be their favorite tactic.

In the end, I decided the VBAC was happening with or without their support. When I showed up at the hospital, all I needed was someone to catch the baby and handle any emergencies. I would also have my doula with me. I was appalled by the fear they instilled in their patients when they should be empowering pregnant women and encouraging the inner strength we all possess. We were created to give birth and we are capable. If labor goes smoothly, it happens naturally. It is not something to be feared but a wonderful experience that creates the miracle of life. It also creates a mother and a father, a sibling, and a family.

I was able to achieve my goal of a natural birth! It was the single most amazing and beautiful experience of my lifetime. I was blessed and lucky to give birth to my little girl with no intervention. I don't normally brag, but my doula was extremely impressed with how I took command of the birthing room and my own labor experience. I didn't allow them to bully or push me into anything that I wasn't comfortable with or that wasn't necessary to have a safe birth. I was forever grateful to my doula for being there with me and supporting me every step of the way. I will forever be a champion of doulas!

Our second little miracle came into this world premature and required a stay in the NICU. Having a child in the NICU was a trying experience and something I will never forget. We took her home, happy and healthy, nine days later.

Her follow-up exam with an LLMD went smoothly, and she was determined to be a healthy baby. No treatment was necessary.

46

Parenthood and Chronic Illness

THE FIRST FEW YEARS AS parents were truly remarkable. Despite suffering from exhaustion as all parents do, every day was an adventure and a blessing. Something as small as tummy time and a walk with Mom was enough to fill my day with love, purpose, and excitement. My health also seemed to remain intact, and no old symptoms crept into my life. John and I had built a beautiful family with two delightful, perfect little girls. We had so much fun with them.

We enjoyed the little things such as when our oldest, Marie, would laugh at the dog wagging its tail or when John crunched down on a potato chip. Our youngest, Katie, lifted her head at a young age and crawled before we were ready! The sisterly bond between our girls was so astonishing that it took my breath away and warmed my heart. I had never witnessed anything like it. The instant connection they had right from the moment they met was the most beautiful bond I'd ever seen. As they grew, both were considered healthy and thriving—a relief to a mother who had experienced much sorrow and sickness already.

I became comfortable in this new stage of my life and in the role of motherhood. I was happy and soaking up every moment. John was an excellent father, and I adored watching him with our girls. They loved him, loved each other, and loved me. I let life surround me with love and I let my guard down.

If there was one thing I could go back and tell myself during that time, it would be to never let your guard down. It is imperative that we listen to our bodies and take care of ourselves because if we don't, things can happen, and they will.

As our family grew, our home felt smaller. In addition to our children, we had Rock, our 130-pound Rottie/German Shepherd mix, and three cats. The dog and the baby swing alone took up the entire living room. We were on top of each other, and it was time to move. We packed up the house and moved thirty minutes away to a larger home with more space for everyone. With a baby on my hip and one in my arms, I moved our family to start another new chapter.

The timing of the move was challenging with two small children, but maternity leave gave me time to pack. Just two months after moving, I was to return to my job. I dreaded leaving my babies again as all mothers do when maternity leave comes to an end.

Being a full-time working mother with an infant and a toddler proved to be more difficult than I had imagined. I had underestimated how hard it would be on my body. With two toddlers who rarely slept through the night, lack of sleep remained an issue.

I had no time for self-care as weekends were full of laundry and cleaning with one baby on each hip. I was working, cleaning, cooking, doing laundry, scheduling doctors' appointments, paying bills, taking care of the pets, and taking care of the responsibilities we all have to run a household and take care of our families. Life also comes with ups and downs, twists and turns, heartache, and happiness. The emotional stress, good and bad, that comes with these ups and downs plays a role in our health.

One year after returning to work, I suffered great loss when my grandfather and my beloved Rock passed away in the same afternoon. I received the call about my grandfather when I was in the parking lot of the vet's office. I sat in the car and ugly cried harder than I had in a long time. I cried for days on end and became emotionally and physically exhausted. Grief took a toll on my body.

A few months later, symptoms of poor health returned. I began struggling significantly at home and work, and I knew it was time to go back to the doctor. My boss had called me into his office to discuss the potential of moving me to a different position. I pleaded for him to allow me to stay and only move me if I couldn't complete deadlines in a timely fashion. He was truly a remarkable boss and agreed to the plan.

In the past, I had met all deadlines and I was determined that this time would be no different.

47

Frightening Symptoms

I VIOLENTLY AWAKENED FROM SLEEP with a racing pulse and difficulty breathing. My throat felt tight and my skin clammy. I shook, cold to the bone, and the sheets were wet with sweat. I gasped for air, slowly and eventually taking a few deep breaths. Nausea and stomach pain quickly consumed me, and I made my way to the bathroom. My body heaved with force as I vomited food my body rejected. Sitting on the bathroom floor with my head on the toilet, I felt tears run down my cheeks. Feeling profound emotional turmoil and overwhelming anxiety, I was completely drained of all physical and emotional energy from the violent episode. Once the vomiting finally ceased, I crawled back out to my bedroom and lay flat on the carpet. I was now hot and sweating. My entire body felt tingly, and I knew there was a good chance I was going to pass out. John woke up during all the commotion and came to check on me.

"Babe, are you okay?"

"No, I'm so hot, I can't cool off. I might pass out." I could hardly get the words out as I continued lying on the bedroom floor.

John reached up and flipped on the ceiling fan. Immediately, I felt a nice cool breeze wash over my body. I lay still and didn't move.

"I can't believe it, but that's helping."

I didn't move for several minutes. Slowly, I could feel the tingling subside and my body temperature decrease.

"I'll get you some ice water." John ran downstairs and returned with a cup. I sat up and took a few sips and chewed on some ice.

"I don't know what the hell that was, but it was not enjoyable. I'm completely wiped out."

"Did you eat something bad? Are you sick?"

"I don't know."

These violent and bizarre symptoms continued to happen to me often, but only at night around the same time, between 2:00 and 3:00 a.m. During the day, I suffered from POTS, heat intolerance, Raynaud's, irritability, joint pain, and various additional symptoms. It felt like Lyme disease all over again but slightly different. My Raynaud's had gotten so bad that I was unable to shop in the frozen section at the grocery store. With just a few seconds of contact, my fingers turned white, numb, and painful.

48

The Hamster Wheel

ONCE AGAIN, I FOUND MYSELF on a hamster wheel going around and around from doctor to doctor but getting nowhere. No answers. No closer to wellness. No closer to sanity. No closer to understanding.

I wondered, *Is this Lyme disease? Did the treatment not last, or is this something else?* With no success in mainstream medicine, I returned to the LLMD that had helped me during pregnancy. After a thorough examination and testing, she wondered if gluten may be causing an issue for me. Instead of undergoing Lyme treatment again, she suggested we investigate gluten first. Initial standard testing for a gluten allergy and celiac disease came back negative. Wanting to dig a little deeper, I asked around and learned of a Naturopathic doctor who was able to conduct extensive blood work, which would include checking for gluten intolerance, celiac disease, and various other food and environmental allergies. I had suspected food allergies six years earlier when I was first having health issues, but my primary care physician had dismissed the idea. It had even been suggested by my pediatrician when I was a teenager. This was my chance to examine the possibility.

Sure enough, the blood work of the Naturopathic doctor was extensive and provided valuable information! I was positive for gluten sensitivity and had allergies to wheat, barley, and rye. Once I received these results, I never touched gluten again. I knew in my gut the right thing to do was to cut out gluten immediately. As soon as I left his office, that's exactly what I decided to do. I went completely gluten-free.

The months following this decision were very difficult. Giving up gluten cold turkey could only be compared to giving up sugar or an addictive opioid drug. Every single day I thought about gluten. My body craved it. My body needed it. I was completely naïve about how addicted I was to gluten. Each day I suffered from severe hunger, shakiness, extreme weakness, depression, crying spells, nausea, muscle and joint pain, hand tremors, poor concentration, insomnia, anxiety, and always feeling hot or cold. I was constantly uncomfortable and no matter what I ate, I could not get full. I wondered if going cold turkey had been the right decision. Perhaps I should have taken it slower!

Even though I was suffering greatly, after just a week or two, one positive thing did occur. The violent nighttime episodes disappeared! I wasn't having them anymore. I couldn't believe it. And even though I was hungry and could never get full, my GI problems improved, and my stomach appeared to be much happier. It seemed I had found the answer. It took about six months to feel better and for symptoms to mostly subside, and a full year to feel truly adjusted to a gluten-free life.

One year into the adjusted diet, I no longer felt hungry in the way that I used to. Hunger created a completely different sensation. Previously, while gluten was still a part of my diet, hunger would give me the shakes and I would become "hangry" and irritable. I would feel like I had to eat *now*. Once adjusted to the gluten-free diet, hunger felt like gentle fatigue and low energy. I knew I needed to eat just as a car needs fuel. Food provided energy and sustenance. I could go longer without it and did not develop the shakes or become hangry. However, my energy would decrease further and further without food. The change was drastic, and it was for the better.

As time went on, I discovered new recipes, how to substitute ingredients in existing recipes, and even located gluten-free snack substitutes for things I had given up! I was in a groove and on a roll!

49

Good Health Never Seems to Last

WORK WAS GOING GREAT. I was finally healthy enough and back long enough from maternity leave to interview again for a competitive position. This time, I was selected as the most qualified candidate and received a promotion. The promotion came with a pay raise and increased responsibilities which included managing and mentoring a team of new employees. It was an exciting and fulfilling job and satisfied my need to help others. Switching jobs meant switching desks; I would no longer sit around the supportive group that I had grown to love. Luckily, that is when I met Maggie.

Maggie and I were assigned to work together and lead the team. She was kind, generous, intelligent, and a hard worker who sported a pleasant smile! She knew when to be tough and realistic but was also upbeat and cared about others. We had so much fun and truly enjoyed mentoring each and every person on our team.

Not long after working together, she was gifted the unfortunate opportunity of witnessing my health issues. As I was getting ready for work one morning, I unexpectedly became violently ill with stomach pain and diarrhea. Afterward, I was left with weakness and fatigue. Feeling drained and lethargic, I texted my boss to let her know I was sick and would be running late. Missing work brought additional pressure and responsibility now as my absence directly impacted a team of individuals who counted on me. This seemed like a typical food reaction for me, and I felt confident it wasn't a virus. It had been quite a while since I had reacted to food in such a way, but I wasn't overly worried. I'd had a tomato-based meal the night before, and the acidity was likely the culprit, or so I thought.

I arrived at work and managed to make it to lunchtime. I warmed up my food in the break room microwave and sat at my desk to eat. After just a few bites, I didn't feel quite right. My vision started to tunnel, my body grew hot and tingly, and I knew it was coming. Syncope. My body was giving me just enough time to warn those around me. I banged my fist on my desk and yelled Maggie's name to get her attention. It was all my brain could think to do right before I fell to the ground and lost consciousness. This was the first time I passed out while seated, so my fall to the ground wasn't quite as far.

Awakening from the episode, my eyes partially opened. There was a small crowd surrounding me as my body was half inside my cubicle and half in the aisle. Shivering and shaking, I realized I was freezing. My skin was cold to the touch, and I couldn't stop my body from trembling. Too weak to move, the trembling worsened and remained constant.

"Are you okay? Can you hear me?" Maggie asked. Someone behind her handed her an unopened bottle of water. "Do you want some water? Can you sit up?"

I tried to sit up some and took a few sips of the water that was offered. I immediately lay back on the ground. The rest is sort of a blur. Coworkers surrounded me but only one towered over me as he sat in my desk chair. It was Troy.

We had started working for our employer around the same time and had always thought of ourselves as kindred spirits. Since the day we met, we noticed similarities in our personalities and got along well. There wasn't a bad thing I could say about Troy. We looked out for each other, and he was smart and possessed great integrity. I was out of it but noticed Troy was talking to someone on my desk phone.

As Troy hung up, he said, "I called an ambulance for you, and they are on their way. Is there anyone else you want me to call?"

"My husband. Can you ask him to meet me at the hospital?" I gave Troy his phone number and he took care of it for me. I will never forget what he did for me that day and the kindness that my coworkers showed.

Maggie held my hand, and Troy sat with me until the ambulance arrived. I was taken out on a stretcher and immediately evaluated in the ambulance. My body continued to tremble and shake. Chest pains, weakness, and cold chills persisted. When I arrived at the ER, they gave me medication that made me immediately pass out.

This would not be my only hospital visit as they would continue over the next two years. Reasons for my hospital visits typically included syncope, heart palpitations, or Supraventricular tachycardia (SVTs). On one occasion, I had an SVT so severe while driving during my lunch break that I almost wrecked my vehicle. My heart rate abruptly sky rocked to over 170 beats per minute. My heart felt like a light switch that had been turned on, and then within less than a minute, turned off again. My body remained in a state of alert for hours afterward and my heart rate stayed in the 120s.

From then on, I had anxiety while driving. I was terrified it would happen again and that I wouldn't be so lucky the next time. Work continued to be a struggle. I couldn't get through an entire week, or even an entire day, without feeling symptomatic. I often had to take breaks, use leave, and utilize the Family Medical Leave Act (FMLA) to survive and maintain employment.

At that point, I had been promoted again to management and, unfortunately, no longer had the strong daily support system I once had. The individuals who surrounded me now held me to a higher standard as I was their supervisor. There wasn't a friend in the bunch. Luckily, I continued to maintain great friendships and had mentors outside my unit. My direct supervisor, however, was a character of sorts and completely lacked any ability to manage others. With a unit laden with strong type-A personalities, it was quite a mess when I showed up. Let's just say, I was now a member of the circus, and not the fun kind. It was a circus nobody wanted to be a part of.

I quickly realized some employees had the false impression that I was to be available to them twenty-four-seven. This was certainly not the case. It had also not been my experience on teams I had led and mentored in the past. Perhaps it was my title of supervisor that caused employees to occasionally become frustrated with my absence as if time missed were a crime. The thing is, you never know what someone else is going through. I pushed myself to be present as often as possible and was still working with my doctors to figure out what was causing my symptoms.

Doctors began to suspect that the building I worked in was playing a role in my health. It was known for water leaks, which often occurred directly above the head. Water regularly dripped onto desks and the cloth walls of cubicles before making it to the carpeted floor. Buckets would frequently be seen throughout the building to catch water. There was much talk about mold growing inside the drop ceiling as it had been seen by employees when the tiles were removed to conduct repairs. Two of my coworkers and I sat in an area of the building with a long-term leak and subsequently developed a cough that lingered for years. At times, the cough caused vomiting and even incontinence for some affected.

Over the years, the entire building had become known as the "sick building" to the employees that inhabited it. Plagued with mysterious rashes, fatigue, GI issues, recurrent sinus infections, bloody noses, dizziness, and violent coughs, employees often felt unwell, particularly in the garage area. Maintenance joked about the HVAC filters rarely being changed and how the AC units on the roof frequently malfunctioned. The deficient ventilation system did not allow for adequate fresh air, proper air volume, or temperature balancing. Walking through the building, you'd hit pockets of hot air and then enter a frozen tundra. Inconsistent temperatures remained a complaint for decades.

The building was sizable with high ceilings (like Sam's Club or Costco) and fluorescent lighting except for the large garage with the drop ceiling. There was no escaping the bright lights that beat down on you every day, causing migraines, eye fatigue, blurry vision, dizziness, and other symptoms. It was a maze of cubicles with various walkways among them and one long hallway that led to conference rooms.

When I would attempt to walk down that long hallway, there was something about the busy blue carpeting and fluorescent lights that made everything worse. Frequently, I'd have to stop halfway to a meeting to sit and manage my dizziness. Symptoms came and went throughout the day, and I never knew when they would strike. It was especially embarrassing when I would get SVTs or other severe symptoms which would require me to walk out in the middle of meetings.

When I wore a heart monitor as an accessory, it was easy to explain, but nobody knew the extent of what I went through each day. A few times, I had to get out of my desk chair and lay on the floor for a while due to my POTs. That wasn't the first time for me, as it had been a frequent occurrence years prior. It was easier back then when I was surrounded by my great friends Melanie, Laura, Kate, and Tracy. I missed my support network!

For each of the episodes that led me back to the ER, the hospital staff chalked it up to POTs and gave me IV fluids. Once my heart rate returned to normal, they patted me on the head and sent me on my way. However, I would later discover there was a piece of the puzzle all doctors were missing.

What did it take to discover this missing piece? An excellent doctor, of course. At one ER visit, I got lucky. There was an amazing, inquisitive, compassionate doctor on call. You never know what you're going to get at the ER. It's just the way it goes. Each visit is the luck of the draw. This doctor took his time going over my blood work and history and noticed something was off. Mind you, I had been to the ER dozens of times over the last decade, and nobody had ever noticed it.

My potassium was low. Not extremely low, but low at 3.2. Potassium should be anywhere from 3.5 to 5.2. The doctor indicated that I had a history of low potassium and diagnosed me with hypokalemia. He gave me several potassium pills and told me it was imperative that I follow up with my doctor as hypokalemia is a life-threatening condition. If left untreated, it can lead to cardiac arrhythmias and respiratory muscle paralysis.

"Worldwide, approximately three million people suffer sudden cardiac death annually. These deaths often emerge from a complex interplay of substrates and triggers. Disturbed potassium homeostasis among heart cells is an example of such a trigger."[23] Electrolyte imbalances, like potassium, can lead to coma or death.

By 2017, I was diagnosed with a laundry list of medical conditions in addition to Lyme disease and co-infections. For some of them, the cause was unknown (such as hypokalemia).[24] For others, mold illness was suspected. Mold can cause extreme inflammation, further weakening the immune system. For someone with Lyme disease and an already weakened immune system, this can make for a highly dangerous combination. The connection and impact between having both Lyme disease and mold illness is a vast topic that is worth researching, particularly if you are not improving with Lyme disease treatment alone or if you have unexplained health concerns. My LLMD conducted a nasal swab to test for mold illness—which was negative. Due to the results, I had no way of knowing if she was correct, and I moved on with my life as best I could.

Most of the time, I was able to get my medical conditions under control enough so I could function and work full-time. I wasn't doing a great job at it, but I was trying. I continued to utilize FMLA to get me through the tougher days. I had learned to function in the world at about seventy percent or less, depending on the day. I never felt great, and I had learned to push through and make it work. I hid my symptoms as best I could. With two small kids at home, a husband, a career, and a household to manage, I didn't feel like I had any other choice.

In 2020, when COVID hit, I would finally pay the price for this, but we're not quite there yet.

---

[23] Keld Kjeldsen, Hypokalemia and sudden cardiac death, *Exp Clin Cardiol 15*, no. 4: Winter 2010: e96-e99. PMCID: PMC3016067. PMID: 21264075. https://t.ly/4EQac.
[24] Ibid.

50

Mast Cell Activation Syndrome (MCAS)

IN 2018, I JOLTED AWAKE from a deep sleep choking and gasping for air. Grabbing my throat, I attempted to swallow and take deep breaths but was unable. It was difficult to swallow and I couldn't understand why. Anxiety and panic consumed me, and my lips felt tingly and swollen. Finally, I felt relief when I was able to swallow and take a couple of shallow breaths. *What was happening? Why had these episodes returned?* These nighttime episodes were traumatizing the first time around, and I was devastated at their violent return.

Intense nausea and stomach pain took over my body. Overcome with profound weakness, I crawled to the bathroom and lifted myself onto the toilet. Diarrhea followed and then vomiting. I grabbed a trash can as fast as I could and spent the next twenty minutes in the bathroom at the mercy of my body. Once it was over, I crawled back to my bedroom carpet and lay flat on my back, hot, sweating, and on the verge of syncope. These violent episodes were hands down the most terrifying symptom I had experienced to date. I felt confident I had solved this issue by eliminating wheat, gluten, barley, and rye and now it was back. Why?

I returned to my LLMD in search of answers. While in her office, she noticed a rash on my chest and arm. She told me that based on the symptoms I described, and the rash, she believed I had Mast Cell Activation Syndrome (MCAS). The violent nighttime episodes were anaphylactic or pre-anaphylactic reactions caused by MCAS.

What? Anaphylactic reactions? Don't those kill you? I felt like I was dying, but I didn't realize there was an actual risk of that truly happening.

I was overwhelmed by what she was telling me. Within a matter of minutes, two new medical terms were used to describe my symptoms—MCAS and anaphylactic reactions. I may have been overwhelmed, but I felt very confident in my doctor. In all the time I spent with her over the years, she had a record of being correct ninety-nine percent of the time. Not only was she intelligent and accurate, but she regularly displayed nothing but kindness and empathy. Always taking the time to get to know her patients and what makes them tick, she had become my voice of reason and a truly sympathetic ear.

She immediately began scribbling down treatment recommendations so we could work on alleviating symptoms. We scheduled a follow-up appointment to further discuss MCAS and what it meant for me.

Just weeks into treatment, my nighttime episodes disappeared. They were gone! I couldn't believe it, the treatment was working! The doctor was still batting ninety-nine percent, and I was thankful she had noticed that rash! While the nighttime episodes had disappeared, I was still dealing with a variety of other symptoms and frequent visits to the ER continued.

During future appointments, we discussed the fact that the exact cause of MCAS was unknown, but we knew it could be from dysregulation of the immune system caused by Lyme disease and potential mold exposure, or likely both. She was adamant that I was exposed to mold within the workplace and wanted me to find a new job. This was a job I had worked so hard to maintain over the years; it paid well. It was what provided health insurance and income for our family, both of which we desperately needed. I felt stuck, trapped, and unsure since the nasal swab test had come back negative for mold. I proceeded to go to work while undergoing treatment for MCAS.

In the meantime, I once again hit the books. I found mast cells to be a fascinating topic, discovering that they could be both your friend and your enemy. How was that possible?

Mast cells are the gatekeepers of our bodies that assist in protecting us against unwanted visitors. Keeping watch, they fight off infection and heal wounds.

When someone has Mast Cell Activation Syndrome, it causes their mast cells to react inappropriately by recognizing benign items as unwanted visitors and attacking them. The mast cells devise frequent attacks on various substances or products we are exposed to such as high-histamine foods, alcohol, beauty or healthcare products, environmental stimulants, chemicals, mold, temperature, barometric pressure, storms, medication, and much more. In fact, when patients become aware of their MCAS diagnosis and begin to track and observe, they may discover they have thirty or more various individual triggers. That is a lot of enemies for one body to potentially encounter throughout the day.

Mast cells have also been known to contribute to "a number of other inflammatory and autoimmune conditions, such as rheumatoid arthritis, inflammatory bowel disease, and multiple sclerosis." ... It has even been shown "that mast cells within the microenvironment of certain cancers may even promote tumor formation and growth."[25] There was still much research needed in the area of MCAS, as it has just received a diagnostic code on October 1, 2016 referring to it as, "D89.4 Mast cell activation syndrome and related disorders."[26] This does not mean that's when MCAS was first discovered, but when it first received a diagnostic code. "These codes facilitate patients getting insurance coverage, applying for disability, and obtaining the medications they need. They also enhance recognition of these diseases and increase their credibility."[27] Since there was still very little recognition and resources regarding MCAS, I relied upon the knowledge of my LLMD as well as what I could find online and in books.

The second step in my treatment journey, after trying the medications suggested by my LLMD, was to adjust my diet. Those

[25] Cliff Takemoto, Mast Cells—Friend or Foe? *Journal of Pediatric Hematology/Oncology 32*, no. 5 (July 2010): 342-344. DOI: 10.1097/MPH.0b013e3181d9da79, https://t.ly/ipIpS.
[26] "2024 ICD-10-CM diagnosis Code D89.4: Mast Cell Activation Syndrome and Related Disorders," ICD10Data.com, Accessed October 17, 2023, https://t.ly/fXdIv.
[27] "ICD-10 Codes," The Mast Cell Disease Society, Accessed October 17, 2023, https://t.ly/HB8OQ.

with MCAS must avoid foods that are high in histamine or histamine liberating. This was far more complicated than a gluten-free diet or even the Lyme disease diet I had had in the past. First, I had to learn what it all meant. What is histamine? What is histamine liberating? What foods are high in histamine? Could I react to foods that *aren't* high in histamine? What foods were safe for me? Did I also have Histamine Intolerance? Histamine Intolerance is "a disorder associated with an impaired ability to metabolize ingested histamine."[28] What did it all mean, and where should I begin? This step alone was intimidating.

After much digging, I came upon the website Mast Cell 360 by Beth O'Hara which offered a suitable diet while the Intolerances App (the app with a strawberry symbol) allowed me a method to track foods. This gave me a good starting point and a plethora of information.

This illness quickly became the most difficult to manage while attempting to work full-time. Convenient meal options such as leftovers and takeout from restaurants were eliminated, making meal planning challenging. Foods that were not freshly cooked were considered high in histamine. This is because as food sits in your refrigerator and ages, the level of histamine rises. The same is true for food served in restaurants. There is no way to know how fresh your food is or if it contains other ingredients that you might react to.

In combination with modifying my diet, I continued to take antihistamines (Benadryl and Zyrtec), cromolyn sodium, and diamine oxidase (DAO) before meals daily. It was suspected that I may have a diamine oxidase deficiency, which is an enzyme that helps your body break down histamine from foods. To help my body with the digestion of histamine within foods, I had to take DAO within the first fifteen minutes of a meal. If meals were interrupted, another pill would be required. That may not have been a big deal, except these pills were expensive. Meals had to be

---

[28] Oriol Comas-Basté et al., Histamine Intolerance: The Current State of the Art, *Biomolecules 10*, no. 8, (2020): 1181, DOI: 10.3390/biom10081181, PMCID: PMC7463561, PMID: 32824107, https://t.ly/WJI6X.

planned, and constant interruptions were costly and symptom-inducing.

Meetings, employees, coworkers, my boss, and all the responsibilities that come with working disrupted my meal schedule and my ability to take care of myself properly. My inability to control my environment (air quality, room temperature, the scent of perfume wafting by, etc.) caused my body to erupt in fury. Rashes, sensitivity to heat, weakness, migraines, SVTs, heart palpitations, and various other symptoms plagued my body. Due to my work circumstances, symptoms continued no matter what I did, despite some improvement.

After a few months of treatment, the rashes became so prominent that I was getting stopped by coworkers. They would even call others over and suggest we go outside to take photos for my doctor. I felt like I had suddenly become a circus sideshow! "Hey everyone, come over here! Check out Kristin's rash!" The rash was a visible indicator of how I felt, but nobody knew what it was like to live inside my depleted body.

51

COVID-19

ON MARCH 17, 2020, EVERYTHING changed. That morning, I dropped the kids off at school like any other day. However, instead of heading straight to work, I zipped over to the grocery store on the hunt for chicken. Chicken was a necessary staple in my diet, one which I relied upon heavily, and it was disappearing from the shelves! I tried not to panic, but I had made finding chicken a priority.

I snagged what I could find from the shelves (which wasn't much) and took it home to place in the freezer. After checking it off my list, I resumed my route to work, feeling a pit in my stomach that I shouldn't be going at all. Upon arrival, I explained the reason for my tardiness but it seemed nobody comprehended the gravity of the situation for me. Without chicken, my diet would be very limited. This could put me in a position of having to eat something that would send me spiraling into a sea of symptoms.

By that afternoon, we were informed that the school systems as well as my government employer were closing. At first, it was alarming, causing the world to feel uncertain. On the other hand, it was exciting to be let out of work early. The world had already changed, impacting so many, including myself. Everyone was flustered and entering the unknown.

So, what did we do?

Bought toilet paper of course! As soon as I was released from work, I was on my second hunt of the day! Who would have thought that would be a thing? Toilet paper was flying off the shelves and none could be found.

Since I was still kid-free for the afternoon, now was my chance. I headed over to the CVS down the street, which permitted the purchase of one four-pack per person. That was not going to be enough for two grown adults and two small children, one of whom used an inappropriate amount no matter how many times I explained that a few squares would do. Dashing over to Walgreens next, I was able to purchase another small four-pack. Feeling successful in my mission, I headed over to the school to pick up the girls.

The days that followed were stressful and uncertain. COVID-19 was spreading, and everything was closing. Restaurants, stores, bowling alleys, theaters, schools, and various other establishments closed with no indication as to when they would reopen. Folks were sent home and told to stay there, avoid others, and only go out if they had to. If you did venture out, you were asked to wear a mask, the only protection we had against the virus at the time.

The girls were supposed to perform in their very first talent show on stage at school, and both were very excited. We had purchased a fold-up indoor gymnastics bar so they could practice their routines. I sat on the living room floor, recording their practice sessions while simultaneously listening intently to the news. Then I heard it…

…*This just in, folks… All schools will be closed beginning March 18, 2020, indefinitely until further notice…*

"What did they say, Mommy?" Marie asked. "Schools are closed?"

"What about our talent show?" asked Katie.

I saw the looks of disappointment on their faces, and this was only the beginning of what was to come.

52

April-May 2020

OVER A MONTH WENT BY with no word on a return date for school or my job. I decided to pull the girls from daycare but begged them to hold our spots. With the increase in daycare prices due to COVID, it didn't make sense financially to continue to pay for an expensive service that wasn't being utilized. With no school, work, or daycare, this provided the girls and I with an opportunity to spend more time together, which was about the only positive thing we had going for us.

The days and weeks dragged on, the toilet paper shortage became a toilet paper war, and food remained scarce. We finally received word that school would remain closed for the remainder of the year, but that work would be sent home with the expectation that parents would complete it with the children.

It was a little concerning that my youngest wouldn't have the opportunity to finish kindergarten, and that my oldest would never get the one-on-one assistance in math I had requested. Now, it was up to me to finish the year. I had zero teaching experience, except for one year when I worked at a daycare. I would hardly call that experience. Mentoring and training grown adults at work didn't seem like the proper qualifications.

Despite my total lack of confidence, I jumped from mom mode to teacher mode and did my best to continue their education. We read books each day, completed assignments I came up with, and spent time outdoors. I didn't realize at the time that what I was doing would be considered homeschooling. We were doing just that, and it was fun.

Unfortunately, it wasn't quite enough to keep us occupied all day. I was used to working full-time, so I grew bored. Not knowing what to do with myself, I took on several home projects. I painted and redecorated our living room, painted the girls' bathroom, installed a tile backsplash in the kitchen, cleaned out the outside dryer vent, and completed other projects I never would have considered or had the time to do previously.

By late May, I received a call from daycare and was informed our spots had been filled. Due to COVID restrictions, the classroom ratios had changed and there was no longer room for my daughters. This was incredibly frustrating and disappointing. I had searched everywhere for quality, convenient daycare that could bus our kids to and from school, and this was our only option. Now it was gone.

53

June-December 2020

WITH ONLY ABOUT FORTY-EIGHT HOURS advance notice, I was told I would be required to return to work. This was nearly three months after we originally closed. We no longer had daycare for the children, and I was at a loss for what to do. We had one family member and one friend who stepped up to watch the children two to three days a week. As for the other two days, I was forced to use my leave. Due to the chaos of COVID, I had placed my health on the back burner as I navigated the new issues on my plate. I consulted with my doctors and let them know I would be returning to work. They advised me that I would be considered high-risk during the pandemic due to my health conditions. This had me on edge.

Now I had multiple issues at play. First, we were without daycare. Second, I did not have enough leave to sustain this arrangement long-term. Third, I was forced to return to work among hundreds of people with zero accommodations or consideration of my health conditions. I immediately requested (at my doctor's suggestion) to work nights and weekends to avoid people, but was denied. It became quite clear early on that I was stuck, and that no one was coming to my rescue. There wasn't a single person who could help me navigate the situation, and my employer would be of no assistance.

John decided that he had to do something to help take some of the pressure off me, so he filed for FMLA at work. This allowed him to take me to doctors' appointments and reduced his exposure to COVID-19 for my protection. His boss was not happy about it. He continually reminded him what a burden it was to have to rearrange the schedule weekly to accommodate him and how unfair it was to the other employees. After a few months, his employer terminated his ability to utilize FMLA. My full plate returned once again.

Even though my health and safety were at risk, the world continued to expect the same from me. In fact, it expected even more. My plate was jam-packed to maximum capacity, but the world didn't care.

Parents were screwed.

High-risk individuals were screwed.

The world was not prepared for a pandemic as no provisions or protections were put in place. Everyone at work was still operating in the same manner, sitting in cubicles side-by-side and having in-person meetings. The only change was the poorly fitted masks that most people didn't wear correctly, if at all. Every day I wondered what world I was living in because this world certainly hadn't adjusted or assisted this high-risk mother of two. I was left to figure it out on my own.

Work went on like this for a few months until I took matters into my own hands by filing a reasonable accommodation. It took me a little while to discover that this was the proper route and to get the paperwork filled out by medical professionals. This finally allowed me to work nights and weekends! It also eliminated the need for family and friends to assist (who were not available long-term) and reduced my risk of exposure to COVID-19.

Working evenings allowed me to step in and assist other units on projects and deadlines when needed. I was able to pick up where they left off when they headed out for the day. I loved being helpful to those who truly appreciated it and could use the helping hand. I was recognized for my efforts, but it's not why I did it.

On my way to work one evening right around the Christmas holiday, I called to check on my friend and former cubicle neighbor, Melanie, only to discover that she was still at work. Stressed to the max and short-staffed, she was working hard to meet a deadline. Due to Covid protocols, staff were often out on quarantine, adding complexity to managing office staff and accomplishing work tasks. Hearing the distress in her voice, I immediately changed course and drove to our second office location. I no longer worked in that building and had been moved to our new facility.

Working alongside Melanie was fun and felt like old times. It lessened the stress of the night for both of us. Sometimes all it takes is someone who cares about you to join you down in the trenches. We were the only two people working in that area of the building that evening, so it couldn't get much more COVID-safe than that.

After working hard for about an hour, Melanie looked over at me, her face wrinkled with confusion, "Did you notice that rash on your chest and arm?"

"What?"

"Look down at your arm and at your chest there," she said, pointing at me.

I looked down. Sure enough, there was a rash.

"Huh," I said with a shrug. "I'm not sure why I have that." I opened my lunchbox and pulled out a turkey sandwich on gluten-free bread.

"Are you supposed to be eating that?" Melanie inquired as I bit into it. "I thought you weren't supposed to eat lunch meat?"

"I'm not, but it's getting harder and harder to manage this schedule, so I just grabbed this on my way out."

"Look at your rash now!" Melanie gasped.

It had grown to about twice the size and was spreading up my neck and down my arm.

"It's probably this damn building combined with my choice of dinner. My body doesn't like it."

We were sitting in the garage area of the building where the ceiling was suspected of having mold. Typically, I'd break out in hives as soon as I entered that area. Employees had commented on it daily in the past. Thankfully, our unit no longer sat back there as we had been relocated to the new facility as soon as we returned to work in June. I hadn't set foot there in a while, not until that night.

I don't know why I hadn't thought of the mold when I arrived, most likely because I was focused on helping a friend and a unit that had given much to me in the past. I also had so much on my plate that my health was never my first consideration anymore.

The school year was underway and the girls had been enrolled in virtual school. This was a new experience for us. As the school year approached, there was much talk about the potential for virtual school, and John and I ultimately decided it was what was best for our family.

Virtual school ended up putting a lot of unanticipated responsibility on me. Every day, I woke the kids up early and got them ready to be on camera with their teacher and classmates. Getting the children ready for school was nothing new, but how the rest of the day followed was.

Every day as soon as school concluded (between 3:45 and 4:30 p.m. due to the chaos) I cleaned up schoolbooks and materials, washed lunch dishes, and got ready for work. I prepared and cooked fresh food for dinner (because of my specific diet) and headed out as soon as my husband arrived home.

I rarely worked past midnight since I had to turn around and wake the kids up for school each morning. I didn't want to add a lack of sleep to the mix as my health conditions never fared well under those conditions.

John did not have a flexible job and having him help wasn't an option for us. His boss had made it very clear that no additional accommodations would be made for him. School took place during the day, and he couldn't be home during those hours. Instead, he took the evening shift—preparing dinner each night and getting the children ready for bed. It wasn't an easy task as they were used to having Mom tuck them in. Some nights when I arrived home from work, they would sneak out of their rooms to greet me at the door.

As time went on, I quickly realized that virtual school was some form of hell that I had traveled to during COVID-19. This mode of education did *not* work for a first grader, a third grader, or our family. I ended up doing most of the teaching myself. My youngest became overstimulated by all the little voices talking at once and the chaos that came with attempting virtual school at that age. Children ran around during instruction not paying attention, bringing toys to the computer like it was show-and-tell time, had loud animals in the background, spun around in their chairs, you name it. We even witnessed several uncomfortable situations with parents yelling in frustration and throwing schoolbooks, half-naked family members walking by, and overheard conversations.

I cried every single day for a month. Virtual school was emotionally exhausting. It became harder and harder to get my kids online at the appropriate times or to get my youngest to sit for her weekly spelling tests (which she dreaded). My oldest would test my patience by turning off her camera and refusing to participate. I was ready to pull out my hair! On top of that, I had to go to work in the evenings when I was already exhausted and completely drained from the day.

My role at work continued to be that of a supervisor, managing a team of people. Since I was now working evenings and weekends, I wasn't there at the same time as my employees (except for a few), and I was slowly losing control due to a lack of support. I was still available by phone or e-mail during the day if my employees needed anything, and I did see a few of them every evening. Despite that, my direct bosses refused to include me on important matters, and it became increasingly difficult to manage while on another shift.

When the pandemic began, my direct boss dropped our unit like a hot potato, leaving us in the wind to fend for ourselves. I stepped up and ensured everyone remained informed and ran the unit on my own. It was as if everyone had forgotten my efforts and all I had done to help those around me, including other units. Now, there I stood in need of support and nobody came. If I had had support, it may have worked out, but we were all just trying to survive the pandemic. I was out of sight, out of mind to them, and nobody seemed to care why I wasn't there. Instead, they became frustrated with me. We changed bosses a few times along the way, and each of them involved me to varying degrees, some better than others.

Empathy and compassion were not generously given at work. The schedule became more difficult to maintain, and my eating habits declined. I would grab what I could at work for dinner. One example being the evening I brought the turkey sandwich. Deli meat is a *huge* no-no on a low-histamine diet. It was the equivalent of inviting anaphylaxis to come knocking at my door, especially with the combination of mold exposure.

I was numb to my life and moving through the motions just trying to survive. What I ate and how I felt were no longer my priority. Instead, it was simply getting through the day and meeting my obligations so the kids got an education, and I received a paycheck.

54

January 23, 2021

I OPENED MY EYES SLIGHTLY and peeked at the digital clock on my bedside table. Eight o'clock, ugh! I don't want to get up. I rolled over, pulling the covers up to my neck. A sliver of light snuck through the blinds and hit me right in the face. I squeezed my eyes shut and rolled over again, nestling my cheek against the soft fleece blanket. Feeling warm and cozy in my soft bed, I let out a sigh of reluctance about beginning my day. It was Saturday, and I didn't have to work until later that night, so what was the rush? I finally had some time for myself.

"Moooommmm, are you up?" Katie yelled from the hallway.

The kids were up. I could already feel the me-time slipping through my fingers. "I guess I am," I replied.

I stretched out my legs and arched my back, attempting to wake up for the day. I immediately noticed something wasn't right. My legs didn't feel the same.

My legs. I can't feel them.

My legs. Wait, I literally can't feel them! How is this possible?

Okay, don't panic.

I sat up slowly and started rubbing each leg. Perhaps they were asleep?

Huh? My arms feel strange. Why is it so difficult to rub my legs? Oh my God, it's in my arms too. Why are they tingling? Are they asleep too? I used one arm to reach over and rub the other arm. Okay, why is this so hard to do?

I outstretched both arms, attempting to move my body around, and winced in pain. *What is that pain in my back? Is it my trap muscles, my spine, or both? I can't tell where this pain is coming from.* As I observed the discomfort in my back, I noticed the same strange numbness and tingling in my back up my skull. *What the hell?* I tried to swing my legs over the side of the bed and stand up. I couldn't do it. Why was it so difficult to move?

"John, wake up." I tried not to panic as I attempted to wake my husband. He stirred a little. "John, wake up!" I said a little louder.

"What? What's going on?"

My voice quivered. "I... I don't know. I can't feel my body."

"What do you mean?"

"I don't know."

John opened his eyes slightly and looked at me. "What do you mean you don't know?"

"It's everywhere. I thought it was just my legs, but it's everywhere."

"What's everywhere?"

"Numbness and tingling."

John sat up, rubbing his eyes.

"I just woke up. I'm still trying to figure it out. I don't think I can walk. I can't feel my legs, and I have numbness and tingling in my arms too, and up my back and skull."

"Maybe your body just fell asleep. Move around and try to wake it up," he said.

"I don't think that's it. I thought that at first about my legs, but it's not going away."

John was fully awake now. "Let's try to get you up." He came over to my side of the bed and helped me swing my legs over the side. I tried to stand and immediately fell onto John. "What the fuck?" said John.

"Okay, this is not good," I replied.

"Okay, sit back down. Let's give it a few minutes."

I sat on the bed and waited. Slowly, I could feel a slight change in sensation. I tried to stand again, and I was able to, but I could only take a few steps with extreme difficulty. John helped me get dressed, and we contacted the on-call doctor for my PCP's office.

"Kristin, you need to go to the hospital immediately. We don't know what this is, and you could become paralyzed," she said.

"Paralyzed?" I exclaimed.

I know doctors are supposed to encourage you to go to the hospital when there is cause for concern, but those words were not reassuring. Did she have to mention becoming paralyzed? Could she have perhaps rephrased or used a calming tone? Maybe she felt it best to clearly state the gravity of the situation. Tears immediately poured down my face in fear and confusion. I called my local PCP directly for a second opinion.

"Hi, Kristin! What's going on?" asked Doctor Rosewood.

"I'm sorry to bother you. I know you're not on-call tonight."

"It's all right, Kristin. Tell me what's going on."

"Honestly, I don't know. I woke up with numbness and tingling all over my entire body."

"You woke up like this?"

"Yes."

"Any other symptoms?"

"Yeah, actually. I have awful pain in my back, and I'm dizzy and fatigued. I feel like my blood pressure must be off. It also hurts to touch my skin."

Doctor Roosewood responded in a calm and soothing voice, "Okay, well what I would suggest is that you go ahead and head to the hospital to get checked out."

Sometimes all it takes is a calm tone of voice and a little reassurance to make a patient feel better. That's exactly what I got from Dr. Roosewood. She had a calm nature and truly cared about her patients. She always took time with them and was there when we needed her.

Now, I know it seems like an obvious choice to head to the ER with an issue like this suddenly appearing, but I was still processing what was happening. I needed to hear the voice of a doctor I could trust and have them confirm my concerns. We were also in the middle of a pandemic and the hospital was the last place I wanted to go to.

John called his mother and asked her to come by to watch the children for us, and we headed to the emergency room.

The emergency room was surprisingly quiet, and we were taken back quickly. Once I was placed in a room, a nurse began to administer an IV for fluids and blood work while another entered data into a computer.

As the nurse was placing the IV, I looked at her perplexed, "I can't feel the needle at all."

"What do you mean, sweetie?" she asked.

"I can't feel that needle. The numbness is too strong I guess."

The two nurses exchanged concerned glances across my hospital bed.

"Okay, you may want to hide your concern right now!" I said. The look they gave each other is one I'll never forget. In all my visits to the ER, I had never seen concern like that on the faces of the nurses.

The nurse rubbed her gloved hand along my forearm. "Can you feel this?"

"No, not really. It just hurts when you do that. My skin burns. All I feel is pain instead of the normal sensation when someone touches you."

The nurse continued to place the IV. Once she was done, she motioned for the other nurse to follow her out to the hallway. "We will be right back, sweetie. We are going to consult with the doctor."

With that, the nurses vanished. I leaned back in the hospital bed, in my hospital gown, once again surrounded by the familiar sounds and smells. I could hear chatter in the hallway, see nurses scurrying by, hear the sound of the equipment in my room (especially the blood pressure cuff each time it kicked on), and smell that sterile hospital smell. I swear, each time I visited the hospital the smell was stronger. You become engulfed in it almost immediately and it's in your hair, on your hands, and temporarily burned into your nostrils.

John sat in a chair beside me, nervously shifting his weight. This was a bad one. I knew it. He knew it. I could feel it. This ER visit was different. It was worse. My body had done it this time.

The nurse came back and explained that the doctor wanted to conduct some testing and had ordered blood work. We proceeded, but I didn't have high hopes for the visit. Most of the time, the hospital was only useful for determining whether something life-threatening was going on, but they rarely discovered the cause of anything. At the very least, I hoped I could leave with some reassurance that it wasn't anything serious.

Once the results were in, the doctor explained that everything appeared to be normal, with the exception of low potassium. I found that to be very odd since I was already taking quite a bit of potassium daily for my hypokalemia (low potassium). Why was it low?

The doctor completely brushed it off and stated it wasn't concerning. He then went on to say that the neuropathy could be from hypokalemia or Mast Cell Activation Syndrome.

"You have various health issues that could be the cause of this, and it's very difficult to determine which one is the culprit. I would like you to take six potassium pills and then follow up with your primary care physician as well as a neurologist."

The doctor was very nice and appeared to be somewhat familiar with my health issues. However, ER visits can be frustrating for a Lyme patient. Most of the time, you leave just as sick as you were when you arrived and remain scared, alone, and in pain. I never imagined that I would enter a hospital with sudden difficulty walking and an inability to take care of myself, yet I would be sent home with no answers. What the fuck?

John looked at me with a furrowed brow. "I don't understand," he said as he ran both of his hands through his hair and held the back of his head. His right leg bounced up and down furiously. He squinted his eyes and turned away from the bright lights in the room, a sign of a migraine. "They are going to just send you home like this?"

Too subjugated and depleted by the unbelievable terror and discomfort my body was experiencing, I replied, "I don't know, John. I guess so."

55

Stabbing, Shooting, Burning

WITH EACH PASSING DAY, THE neuropathy and paresthesia (burning, prickling, and tingling) intensified as did my other symptoms. Excruciating pain in my back became almost unbearable. My blood pressure was a roller coaster ride, and the constant dizziness was enervating. Frequent syncope and laborious breathing frightened even my children. My temperature sensitivity and Raynaud's were at its worst, and my skin was on fire. Every single day I sat on my couch, unable to move. Stabbing, shooting, burning pain ensued, resulting in a body that was completely intolerable to inhabit.

Alone each day, with only my young children to help me, I crawled to the bathroom and pulled myself up using the counter. Pulling my pants down felt like razor blades scraping burnt skin. I didn't understand how or why my skin was so sensitive and so painful to touch.

Unable to cook, I was at the mercy of my husband to prepare some sort of meal for dinner once he came home from work. It was my only meal of the day. When I did eat, it was uncomfortable as eating caused painful sores in my mouth. I seemed to be reacting to every food I tried. After meals, my lips and underneath my nose would tingle and swell. The space around both of my eyes tingled, burned, and felt cold as if I'd drawn two raccoon eyes using menthol.

I remained in the same position on my couch for days upon days. Unable to focus on anything, all I could do was watch TV. Since I was easily stimulated, I couldn't tolerate overly emotional shows or anything with action, so I settled on watching *The Golden*

Girls. Those wonderful ladies were calming, funny, and soothing for the soul. I watched *The Golden Girls* for weeks on end. My kids began watching the show with me, and we would sing the theme song together. They learned the characters' names and would ask questions. This became the sole thing we were able to do together, but it was something.

Evenings were rough and nights excruciating. By 7:00 p.m. every evening, my legs gave up completely and I was unable to stand. We began going to bed before that time as a family because it was when Mommy was done for the day. The children questioned why we were going to bed so early, and I would simply reply that my body was sick and needed rest. Eventually, they understood that that was when Mommy shut down for the day. At 7:00 p.m. they would ask, "Mommy, are you shutting down now?"

Getting ready for bed was the biggest challenge of the day for me. First, it required the daunting task of stairs which involved crawling or receiving significant assistance to achieve. Secondly, it required bathing. I attempted showers a few times, but it only weakened me, causing inevitable syncope or worsening of neuropathy and pain. The water pressure felt like a million tiny little stinging needles on my agitated skin. Exiting the shower was misery. The change in temperature from the warm shower to the cooler bathroom air caused extreme neuropathy and painful skin sensations. I discovered that plugging in a small heater and warming up the bathroom prior to a shower was helpful, but it wasn't enough to prevent symptoms.

Cool baths became my only option. Unable to lift my arms for very long, my little one (seven years old at the time) would sit on the side of the tub and wash my hair. Possessing a kind and gentle soul, Katie naturally desired to help me in any way she could. She was the type of child who seemed to feel the pain of others and take it upon herself to care for them. Protective, empathetic, strong, and compassionate, she was my little angel.

My youngest child and I had switched roles; she was taking care of me. This was not the way it was meant to be. This became the single lowest moment of my life. I feared she would remember this, and it would cause fear and attachment issues down the road, or even now. I wondered what she was thinking and prayed that things would get better. They had to, right?

After brushing my teeth, I would stand in the doorway of the bathroom holding onto the doorframe, legs bent and quivering. I dreaded each night when the lights went off for many reasons. My eyes now had extreme difficulty adjusting from light to dark. My right eye in particular no longer seemed to have the capability; it felt as if I was only seeing out of one eye. I worried that my eyes were affected and I would lose eyesight. Nights were a scary thing, and so was sleep.

Each evening as I stood in the doorway, my body was done. Going to bed early was a necessity for more than one reason. Not only was my body unusable by that time, but if I remained in bed for twelve hours, I discovered it would give me enough time to get three or four hours of broken sleep.

The paresthesia and neuropathy overtook my body and made it impossible to sleep for any extended period. As if that wasn't enough, the constant back pain was so agonizing that it was hard to think straight and made sleep unattainable. The pain was in the same location that I had experienced a few years before, after the epidural and birth of my first child.

The feeling of fabric against my skin was a constant irritant and caused me to wince in pain. My clothes felt like a prison. I was completely unable to wear a bra, socks, or closed-toed shoes during the day as the pain and discomfort were far too great. Crawling into bed each night, the sheets created the same sensation. To ensure some sleep, I created a routine. Utilizing my adjustable bed frame, I lifted the head of the bed quite a bit and the feet slightly. I slept in an upright position nightly with a heating pad on my back to dull the pain. Compression stockings (an idea provided by Eve) and a pillow between my legs were a must. I made every effort to remain perfectly still to prevent my clothes and sheets from rubbing my skin. If I followed this routine, it allowed me to get a few hours of broken sleep each night.

My body prevented me from getting the deep sleep it needed. Every few hours, I awoke with surges of adrenaline and what felt like histamine coursing through my body at lightning speeds. Falling asleep created this unnerving sensation that felt like a wave of energy. It had an odd familiarity to passing out. I wondered if my body was experiencing total exhaustion or some sort of adrenal dysfunction. Every day, I was afraid to go to sleep and afraid to wake up. Visits to my doctor's office got me nowhere. Initial potential diagnoses were nerve cancer, multiple sclerosis, paresthesia, and idiopathic small fiber neuropathy.

As time went on and the snow began to fall, the kids requested that I partake in our usual winter activities.

"Let's build a snowman, Momma!" Katie exclaimed.

"Come watch me make a snow angel, Mom!" Marie requested.

I stared longingly out the window at the snow-covered landscape. With the outdoors completely enveloped in a white quilt of beauty, the world had become a quieter place. I always loved the peace of this time of year. Not quite sure how to bundle up enough to enjoy it, I decided to make a go of it anyway. I layered myself up like Randy in the movie *A Christmas Story* and headed outside with my children.

Only able to take a few steps, I ambled out into the yard and remained inert. The children laughed and bounced about, jumping in the snow. I closed my eyes and felt the snowfall softly hitting my face. With the world covered in a white fluffy blanket, all sound was dampened, and I felt alone in a magical, peaceful land. Opening my eyes, I scanned our neighborhood and observed the glistening crystal of ice-covered twigs and branches. What a beautiful world snow creates.

After being distracted by the magnificence surrounding me, I returned to reality only to notice that I was quickly tiring and unable to wiggle my toes. It was time to go inside. I motioned to the children and went back inside the house. As I removed the layers of clothing, socks, and boots, I observed that my toes were white and unable to move. I hobbled over to the fireplace, sat on the floor, and placed my feet toward it. As the fire warmed my feet, they turned red and began to burn. My ears, feet, and hands often turned red accompanied by a burning hot sensation. A change in temperature was a guaranteed trigger for this. The fire wasn't working fast enough as I was still unable to move my toes. It was also difficult to tell if it was working well at all since I was already experiencing numbness and tingling. *Wow, this could have been dangerous. What if I had stayed out there longer? Could I have caused further damage?*

I reached for a heated blanket draped over the rocking chair, turned it on, and wrapped it around my feet. During the colder months, Katie loved a soft heated blanket. Luckily, she had left it plugged in! My poor feet were so dry and cracked. I hated the way they looked and what the nerve damage had done to them. My hair was dry and brittle too, and my nails easily split and cracked. I was happy that I didn't have the energy to make it to a mirror because I no longer liked what I saw. As the blanket heated up, my toes slowly improved and I could wiggle them again. The pain wasn't pleasant, but the brief time with my children enjoying the exquisiteness of the snow had been worth it.

After months of continued symptoms, I began to suffer from exhaustion-induced depression. Minimal, broken sleep does not provide the body with what it needs for healing. I had never been so tired in all my life (even after the many sleepless nights that come with having a newborn baby). This was different. This was so much worse. Months and months without sleep impact your ability to focus, think, and reason. I was unable to conduct any mental or physical tasks. I lived minute to minute, trying to survive each one as it passed.

I remained in my spot on the couch, watching *The Golden Girls* and praying that in time, things would change. The rare occasions I left the couch were to attend medical appointments. Doctors had already conducted numerous tests and taken countless tubes of blood, only to get nowhere. What a familiar road I was on. A road of desolation and misery.

However, there was one thing that was different about this experience. I couldn't focus on my medical care the way I had been able to in the past. My brain wasn't functioning properly and couldn't analyze information, process emotion, or make decisions. I found myself sitting at appointments just staring at the doctor, unable to comprehend what they were saying. I couldn't make rational decisions about my own care. That was a scary thing. It made me feel hopeless, helpless, and out of control. As the person who knew my body best, I couldn't help it. Not unless I could improve the brain fog and regain some clarity.

My next scheduled test was the nerve conduction study (a test that evaluates the function of your nerves) to confirm whether I had small fiber neuropathy. I debated whether to go through with it. I was anxious, stressed, and miserable, and it was extremely difficult for me to get around. I had great concern that the test would irritate my nerves. But how was I ever to get answers if I didn't have tests? It had to be done.

I couldn't drive myself, so John had to take off work (yet again) to drive me to my appointment, kids in tow. Due to the pandemic, we had no daycare and school was virtual. Forcibly, doctors' appointments became a family affair. With pandemic concerns at an all-time high, local family members (most of whom were high-risk) didn't want to take any chances so they remained unavailable to help. The biggest issue causing particular concern was John's job. COVID was being passed around like a cold at a toddler's birthday party. Everyone was getting it, and nobody was careful. It was an irresponsible display of selfishness and a lack of concern for the community. Even though the rest of us were home, our family had no desire to take a chance due to John's circumstances. We understood but weren't happy about it either.

John and the girls waited in the car as I entered the neurologist's office for my test. I ambled inside with bent legs, quivering with each step. I was a nervous wreck as my body was an utter disaster. Dr. Ludwig entered the exam room with a smile on his face, as he always did. Even with the mask on, I could see his smiling eyes and knew it was there under the mask.

"How are we doing today, Kristin?" he asked.

"Same," I replied.

"I know it's challenging to have small fiber neuropathy. We will go ahead and get started so we can get you out of here," he said.

Dr. Ludwig proceeded to insert needles, and I felt shocks throughout my nerves. It was uncomfortable for sure, but if it led to any answers, it was worth it. Once the test was over, I was ready to collapse on my couch and rest. Any activity destroyed me physically and mentally for the day and rendered me completely unable to handle another task. Most days, I could only handle one activity or task before I found myself at capacity. Each test thereafter eliminated possible causes but didn't result in an answer.

By this time, I found myself completely unable to assist my children with virtual education, and school became a disaster. My daughters were turning off their cameras or not showing up on time. Teachers were becoming frustrated. In the beginning, it caused me a great deal of stress and worry. I had to quickly learn to let go of this worry and know that my kids would be okay. We would survive this.

Work continued to move forward during the pandemic as if COVID didn't exist. Management became tired of accommodating me and I heard that some employees felt it unfair. *We have returned to normal hours, and she should be here every single day like everyone else*, I knew they were thinking. But I wasn't capable of that. There was so much I wasn't capable of anymore.

The pressure of the world was immense and the pressure on me as a working mother during the pandemic was astronomical. I felt this weight on my shoulders all while wondering if I would ever walk normally again or resume any sort of normalcy within my mind and body. The sensations within my body were becoming more and more unbearable each day.

Was anyone or anything going to save me from this hell I was living? No. I was on my own. Fighting against my own body while simultaneously fighting against the expectations of the world. I knew I was strong; I would figure it out. I had no other choice. The only way out of this was through it.

The treatment that my LLMD had suggested for treating Mast Cell Activation Syndrome (MCAS) was no longer working, and I found myself reacting to medications such as Claritin, Zyrtec, and Pepcid. While she was the doctor who had originally discovered I had MCAS, my body made it clear that an alternate treatment was necessary. I heard about a functional medicine doctor who specialized in MCAS that could potentially help. There were no other doctors in the area who truly specialized in the illness, so I looked forward to giving her office a call. All of this might have stemmed from increased inflammation and MCAS.

During my first appointment, I sat on the exam table so weak that a puff of air could have knocked me down. While testing my muscle strength, she pulled my leg out and told me to try to resist. With one pull she almost slid me clear off the table. She jumped to catch me, completely shocked by what had just happened. I warned her I had no muscle strength, and now she saw it was true!

It was my first experience with a doctor who looked at my body as a whole to investigate a root cause. Was it mold exposure? Probably. This had already been suspected by my LLMD. Was it heavy metals? Perhaps. Was it my gut? That could explain the food sensitivities. Was it autoimmune? Most likely, due to a history of Lyme. Was it genetic? Potentially, as other family members suffered from similar issues. Within a few months, I was officially diagnosed with MCAS through blood work (in addition to my previous clinical diagnosis by my LLMD), and we began new treatment methods. With additional testing, I was also diagnosed with leaky gut and candida.

I reacted to every—single—treatment we tried. It seemed impossible to get my symptoms under control any further. The one thing I had done for my body almost immediately after the increase in symptoms was limit my diet to three single low-histamine foods. I began with chicken, zucchini, and celery.

I had no other choice as I was once again waking up at night gasping for air. My syncope episodes increased, my blood pressure fluctuated daily at dangerous levels, my ability to walk had been compromised, and I suffered from pain and loss of feeling. Once I restricted my diet, I slowly began to experience some improvement after a few months. It wasn't much, but I welcomed any relief I could get.

In addition to my diet, my functional medicine doctor discovered a combination supplement that helped slightly. It included ingredients such as Vitamin C, Riboflavin (vitamin B2), Niacin, Molybdenum, N-acetyl-l-cysteine (NAC), Quercetin, Bromelain, Luteolin, and Rutin. It controlled much of my sinus issues (runny nose, sneezing, watery eyes) as well as feelings of

185

being off-balance or dizzy. I was still tolerating DAO, which I continued to take before meals. This alleviated any stomach trouble like bloating and pain.

Due to my diet and the new supplement (or so I thought), the numbness and tingling became bearable enough to allow me to drive to work again, so I went. When I say bearable, it may not have been bearable for others, as I've always had a high pain tolerance. I was also used to pushing forward while experiencing pain and symptoms. I forced myself to show up for work despite feeling weary, despondent, achy, and uncomfortable. Shaky and feeble, I resembled a bag of bones. Every step was a battle. I tried to hide it. I needed this job. Work was required to support my family so I would work a few nights a week, as my body allowed. Each evening when I arrived, I was greeted by concerned coworkers and some of my own employees.

As I struggled to walk down the hall, I hobbled past the desks of coworkers.

"Kristin, you look tired! Why are you here?" Elli asked.

"You should stay home. Girl, you're crazy coming in here," Natalie offered.

"I need this job, so I keep coming," I responded with a shrug.

From a distance, I saw Gavin get up from his desk and walk toward me. As he approached, I could see the troubled look on his face.

"Why are you walking in here all alone? Can you make it to your desk? Let me help you," he said as he offered me his arm.

I quickly obliged because, let's face it, I needed the help, and I could tell he cared. We slowly walked to my desk, and he helped me get settled.

As I logged into my computer and began to work, thick brain fog prevented me from accomplishing much of anything. Documents and tasks that were once second nature to me felt unfamiliar. My ability to focus and retain information was severely limited. All my thoughts were stuck behind a thick hazy wall, unable to get through. Discouraged and defeated, I accomplished what I could. As a highly analytical person, typically required and capable of accomplishing complex tasks, I felt lost without this ability. It was gone. I was unable to do my job for the first time. Ever.

The severity of the brain fog likely wasn't evident to the coworkers I encountered at night. We mostly chatted socially and occasionally about work matters. A handful of individuals worked nights mostly due to the pandemic, but some were just overworked and felt pressure to stay late to keep up. The ladies and gentlemen who I encountered at night were incredibly kind to me and would never truly understand how grateful I was to them.

As time passed, the neuropathy worsened, causing further nerve damage, decreased muscle strength, and poor balance. I utilized a walker for mobility within the workplace and discovered our building was not handicap accessible (no ramps or automatic doors). When I arrived in the evenings, my coworkers offered to assist me with the door and provided their cell phone numbers in case I needed anything. They were compassionate enough to provide companionship and a few laughs along the way.

I wish I could say I continued to improve over the next few months, but I stayed about the same. With each step, I had to focus on putting one foot in front of the other. My legs and feet didn't feel like they were mine, and it was as if I were present in some borrowed vessel. The single act of taking a step had a completely different sensation. There were days when I would have to stand in front of a full-length mirror and practice walking so my mind could connect to my limbs again.

Tripping became a common occurrence. It was difficult to feel each step or navigate around objects. Most of the time, I tangled up on my own legs or tripped over my own feet. Without help, I fell hard a few times, smacking against the pavement. I developed a fear of being alone and experiencing a traumatic fall.

I don't know what I would have done without my oldest daughter, Marie. On better days when I was able to attend doctors' appointments, she was my saving grace. My children were often in tow due to a lack of daycare and virtual school. At each appointment, I became frustrated with the lack of handicap accessibility. Marie helped me lift the walker over curbs and up any steps I encountered at entrances; both girls opened doors so I could walk through. Getting into offices was tricky, and my ability to balance had decreased quite a bit due to the neuropathy. The girls did a wonderful job helping their mom when Dad had to work. I don't know what I would have done if they had been younger.

Appointments became increasingly frustrating. Not only due to the lack of handicap accessibility but also because of a lack of understanding. It felt as if my doctors were all giving up on me. With each visit, several doctors recommended that I discontinue working and file for disability. Along with that came suggestions to travel to the Mayo Clinic or the Cleveland Clinic. These facilities are not known for being supportive or advantageous for those with Lyme disease and MCAS. I had been down the road of being poked and prodded in the past and I wasn't about to put myself through that unless I knew it would help. I had heard horror stories of those places, of the repeated tests and of being dissected like a lab animal only to be dismissed and labeled as crazy, or worse. No, thank you.

It felt as if they were pawning me off because they didn't know what to do next. I had no desire to travel to either of those places in my condition unless it was my last option. I would have to be on my deathbed. I kept screaming in my head, *No, you figure this out! Try harder!* Feeling unsure what to do next, I applied to the Undiagnosed Diseases Network at the recommendation of one of my doctors but was denied.

I was later referred to a new neurologist for a second opinion and a nephrologist regarding hypokalemia. Both doctors were able to help me in their own ways, and I appreciated it, but neither was the answer to the complicated myriad of daily symptoms I experienced. They were only able to help with a sliver of my problems. A sliver is good, but it's not the whole pie.

It was at the rheumatologist, Dr. Saari, where my health finally took a decent turn for the better. My original neurologist, Dr. Ludwig, referred me to her to dig deeper. She discovered autoantibodies, inflammation, and a connective tissue disorder. Recognizing the severe nerve damage occurring, she indicated that we had to stop its progression and attempt to reverse the damage. I was immediately placed on steroids and hydroxychloroquine.

Terrified and reluctant to take either, I still obliged. I was willing to try anything at that point.

These discoveries, of course, were all tied back to dysregulation of the immune system, MCAS, Lyme disease, and potential mold illness. But at each visit, the rheumatologist denied the connection and repeatedly stated we would never know why this happened to me. It was also unlikely that the neuropathy and nerve damage could ever be reversed, but we would try. I knew why it was happening but didn't argue with her. It wasn't worth the fight when I knew where she stood. I didn't need her acknowledgment, only her help with her slice of the pie. She was a vital part of my team and she was helping me. There was no changing her mind. However, she wasn't completely wrong. It can be very difficult to determine the cause of small fiber neuropathies, but it's imperative that you do.

Small fiber neuropathy (SFN), where small fiber refers to the smallest nerves of our body, affects C nerve fibers, of which there are two types—somatic and autonomic. "Somatic small fibers mediate our sensation of pain, temperature and vibration. The autonomic fibers mediate most of the autonomic nervous system… and go to almost every organ in our body…"[29]

When autonomic fibers are not working properly, "this causes autonomic disorders at the level of the organs. The question is, what causes small fiber neuropathy? This is where the difference can be made. If an underlying cause can be found, particularly a reversible underlying cause, then we can tackle that cause and treat the core problem rather than treating symptoms…"[30] When the core problem is treated, treatment of symptoms is still necessary as one does not exclude the other.

For example, if a vitamin b12 deficiency is treated, you will most likely still need to wear compression stockings. However, the point of treating the core problem is to hopefully prevent further damage to the nervous system. In the best-case scenario, if there

---

[29] Kamal Chémali, "The Quest to Find an Underlying Cause," (lecture, 2015 Dysautonomia International Conference & CME, Washington, D.C.) July 17-20, 2015, Video of lecture, 28:50, https://rb.gy/plgmdn.
[30] Ibid.

are still viable nerves, we can reverse the process. But this does not always happen. Success in finding something reversible is no more than a thirty to fifty percent chance.[31]

The most common cause of SFN is unknown while the second most common is diabetes. Other known causes are impaired glucose tolerance, amyloidosis (rare disease affecting organs), other monoclonal [Multiple Myeloma (blood cancer) or MGUS (a noncancerous condition affecting plasma cells) for example], vitamin B12 deficiency [32] (resulting from absorption issue, vegetarian diet, gastric bypass, etc.), alcohol and toxins (chemotherapy, heavy metals, etc.), ciguatera poisoning (type of fish in the Caribbean), autoimmune diseases, cancer, infections (HIV, botulism, etc.), hereditary causes (HSAN types I to V or HSAN III, Porphyrias, etc.), and paraneoplastic (remote manifestations of cancer such as ANNA (Anti-Hu), Lambert-Eaton Myasthenic Syndrome, or Myasthenia gravis).[33]

Dr. Saari had already tested me for many of those conditions and had placed me on the only medications she thought I could benefit from. Within about four months, the neuropathy began to improve. I couldn't believe it. It slowly dissipated from my skull, my back, and my arms but remained steady in my legs and feet. I could feel my body desperately clawing its way out of the hole it had fallen into.

I can't explain what it was like to finally experience some relief. Any relief. It was at this point (about ten months after the date of the onset of neuropathy and paresthesia) that I finally began to get enough sleep to feel like a sane person again. The crying spells and

---

[31] Ibid.

[32] "In order to determine if you have a b12 deficiency, testing b12 alone is not sufficient. Standard b12 tests will *not* tell you how much b12 is in the cells, and this is what counts. There is no way to measure b12 within the cells, but you can measure other elements of a chemical reaction in which b12 is important. This is methylmalonic acid (MMA) and homocysteine. When b12 is deficient, both of these are going to go very high in the blood. Often, b12 is normal in the blood pursuant to lab standards but you will find that MMA and homocysteine are high, which is evidence of b12 deficiency." Kamal Chémali, "The Quest to Find an Underlying Cause," (lecture, 2015 Dysautonomia International Conference & CME, Washington, D.C.) July 17-20, 2015, Video of lecture, 28:50, https://rb.gy/plgmdn.

[33] Ibid.

the depression began to subside. I still wasn't getting nearly enough rest with only one solid four-hour chunk per night. The remainder of the time was spent awake, tossing and turning, and managing symptoms. It was still a vast improvement from the nonexistent sleep I had been experiencing for months on end. The relief of four straight hours of sleep can only be described as pure bliss.

I was on a low dose of prednisone for a few months, and then only hydroxychloroquine remained. It took eight months before I felt any sort of improvement in my legs and feet, but it eventually came. My blood pressure began to normalize, syncope episodes became less often, and overall, my body felt calmer. Every day was different. Some days I had neuropathy in my skull, back, or arms, but it wasn't constant as it had been before. The neuropathy in my legs and feet remained but it was not as intense. Some days it was replaced by my legs feeling incredibly heavy, as if they weighed five times as much as they had before.

Now and then my body would provide me with a glimmer of hope that I could get better. Sometimes I would even feel normal for an entire hour! But it was always a twisted joke my body played on me because it never lasted.

Despite my improvement, my body remained in shambles. I felt as if I were walking a tightrope and all it would take was one mistake for me to lose my balance and fall. I was completely unable to live a normal life anymore. Without the ability to sleep five to eight hours a night, I wasn't a functioning human. Symptoms remained and I was incapable of getting up for a job each morning, cleaning my house or even vacuuming one room, making meals for my family, or going to the store on my own. I had become dependent on others for help once again, and I was forced to completely change my life to adjust to this new normal.

I returned to my job part-time during daylight hours, working just a few hours at a time, two days a week. Since I would be surrounded by people and a nurse was on staff, the doctor felt better about it but insisted I apply for disability. Each day I worked, I arrived in the parking lot and searched for a handicapped parking space by the front entrance. Working the day shift was frustrating as there were never enough handicap spaces. Most days I'd park elsewhere, such as a space reserved for charging electric cars. There sure were plenty of those, and most were empty! Once I parked and exited my vehicle, I limped back to the trunk to retrieve my walker, my hand gliding along the side of my vehicle for balance. Lifting the walker from the trunk and unfolding it for use was challenging and painful. Not only was it problematic to maintain my balance, but muscle fatigue and weakness made it painful to lift the walker (and this was with a lightweight model).

The entire routine of parking and getting my walker ready took several minutes. Once situated, I pushed my walker toward the front door, passing anyone who was coming or going or sitting outside for a break. Immediately, I observed all eyes were on me. Coworkers couldn't stop themselves from staring at the girl with the walker. When I approached the door at the same time as another person, the reaction of each person differed. Some awkwardly let the door slam behind them, not knowing if they should assist me or not. Others held the door open for me, with their chest puffed out with pride as if they had done me this huge favor because I couldn't possibly figure it out alone. Then there were those who held the door open quietly with a smile. It was a very odd experience, suddenly being thrown into the world of disability culture and being forever changed by it all in a short period.

Have you ever noticed that not all buildings are handicap accessible, even some doctors' offices? Have you ever attended an event and wondered how a handicapped person would fare there? Have you ever taken public transportation, flown on a plane, or vacationed at a beach and wondered what a handicapped person would do with a walker or wheelchair? How would they access these things? Are you aware that not every employer is willing to accommodate someone with disabilities and that they are often seen as a burden?

Everywhere I went, I watched, observed, and noticed things that I hadn't considered previously. I saw the world differently now, and I was saddened. The world is not built for the disabled, nor is it built for inclusion. Why is that? Why are the elderly, the sick, and the disabled tossed aside? It's a systemic issue that cries out for a solution. We must do better for those who are suffering. If you were crossing the street and witnessed a disabled person struggling to do the same, would you assist them? How is this any different? I cried tears of sadness for others, and some for myself too. The disabled deserve to enjoy the beauty of the world and for that world to be accessible whenever possible.

The following school year, the children were officially homeschooled, and I applied for disability retirement with the insistence of my doctors. I resisted the idea for quite a while. Let's face it, since COVID had hit and my health had taken a turn, my job had become completely unenjoyable. As my health diminished, so did my love for my job. It was no longer possible to be the person I had been before—a hard-working, passionate individual determined to make a difference. I was too tired for that now. Too worn out for that now. Too sick for that now.

It was time for me to look out for myself and live a different sort of life: a life full of simple pleasures, nature, and peace with a focus on wellness. Fairly quickly, my disability was approved, and I got my wish. Applying was no easy task. The mountain of paperwork required, as well as the energy it took to gather medical records and fill out forms, was an accomplishment in itself for someone in my physical and mental condition.

A few weeks before the approval of my disability, my functional medicine doctor discovered another MCAS treatment for me to try, compounded Ketotifen. She was following the work of Dr. Afrin, a leading expert in the field, who had found Ketotifen to be beneficial for his patients. When trying something new, MCAS patients often start with a small amount as we tend to have big reactions if we respond negatively. Despite starting low and slow with a quarter of the recommended dose, I experienced a powerful reaction. Almost immediately, I was hit with profound fatigue, the weight of which rendered me incapacitated.

In the days that followed, insomnia, irritability, joint pain, and heart palpitations devoured me. But there was something different about these symptoms. At first, it felt like I was coming down with an illness. An uneasy sick feeling existed in the center of my chest. This medication was severely impacting me. I quickly lowered my dose by cutting it in half as I wanted to give it a fair shot. I had seen too many success stories with this medication not to.

After a little retrospection, I realized that ketotifen was hitting the very heart of the issue. The exact symptoms that I had been suffering from were increasing, but that wasn't all. They were being stirred up. It was as if this medication was attacking and stirring up the very thing inside me that was causing so much turmoil. After a little over a week, the reactions began slowly improving and I started to feel some positive effects. This ended up pushing me forward toward better health. It improved my sleep, slightly increased my energy, provided me with a clearer mind, and diminished my constant suffering from neuropathy. It was certainly not a magic solution, however. I hoped that one existed, but it never came.

In a desperate attempt to regain strength, I tried to get in my pool to exercise. Unbeknownst to me, chlorine can be an MCAS trigger. A pretty severe one at that. The moment I exited my pool, my legs gave out. I wasn't at all prepared for the wobbly jelly-like feeling. Then came the burning. It felt like both of my legs were on fire. I motioned for John to grab the water hose so I could immediately hose off my body. As soon as the water came out I held it over my head like a shower hoping it would wash away the pain and discomfort. Amazingly, it did provide some relief but it took days to recover from one dip in the pool.

This is when I found Qigong. I was determined to move my body, and this seemed like a good fit. In the past, I had enjoyed Zumba and kickboxing. With my body in feeble condition, even my attempts at Yoga were unsuccessful. Just a few poses left me feeling dizzy, off balance, and weak. Qigong, on the other hand, involved gentle movements to improve energy, health, and wellness. At first, I could only manage a few gentle movements at a time, but it was satisfying. It fulfilled a part of my life that was missing, which was my love of exercise.

I continue to fight this battle with my own body, attempting to regain strength and perspective. I try not to look at it as a battle but as a journey of nourishment and encouragement. A time for me to fuel my body and mind with the things it requires, to achieve a more comfortable life. I remain walking this tightrope, trying to stay balanced every day. It's not easy, but they say nothing worth doing ever is.

I have realized many things after decades of following the ebbs and flows of my own health. For one, the world around us moves swiftly and carelessly. We must take time to stand still. Most of us get up early every day and work a job Monday to Friday that we may not like. We aim to please others all day to show them respect and to earn a paycheck. We fall victim to the desires of others and to the countless obligations that require our attention.

Each night, we crash into bed exhausted, without ever getting enough rest to recover from the fast pace of the world. And then what do we do? We get up the next day and repeat. We are bombarded by commercials and social media attempting to sell us products by telling us we need them or aren't good enough without them. Folks regularly compare themselves to others and want more and more. We take care of our families and households and attend our jobs. We are constantly on the move all while being interrupted by text messages, phone calls, social media alerts, meetings, requests, favors, and obligations.

We journey through life only ever pushing pause during the week to potentially take a family vacation, attend a funeral or celebration, or take care of emergencies.

This is all that we pause for.

Why is that?

Why can't we put ourselves first? Why don't we respect ourselves first? Isn't it true that we are supposed to put our oxygen mask on before we put on the mask for others? So, why aren't we doing that? Why can't life adjust to our individual needs and fit around us versus the other way around? Why do we bend over backward to satisfy someone else's narrative as opposed to writing our own?

Living like this was considered normal, and it was time I broke up with normal.

56

Breaking Up with Normal

MY MIND AND BODY WERE crying out for me to live a different sort of life, and so, I intended to do just that. It was time for a shift.

Over the course of my life, I had pursued hobbies, exercised, and squeezed in two family vacations a year. I had also seen my doctors regularly and taken my medications. I had meditated, did Zumba, enjoyed nature, and spent time with my family. Those were all good things, right? Then why was I always struggling at work, feeling sick, and ending up in the ER every year? Why did my health get so bad? Why had it turned into a hellish nightmare this time around?

Because I never put myself first.

I never felt that I could. I had to work to support my family. I can't rely on someone else for support. That's crazy, right? I can't stop and take multiple breaks throughout the workday. That's preposterous. I can't take several days off at a time, turn my cell phone off on vacation, and disconnect from the world without feeling guilty or like I'm missing something. Why not? Seriously, what are we really missing?

I lugged my sick body around through the days and kept going even when it sent warnings not to. I continued to work even when it told me, "Not today!" I exposed myself to a mentally and physically toxic work environment in exchange for a paycheck. Each time I experienced a flare of my health conditions, I rested briefly, returned to the doctor, and pushed through them until the next set came along. Sometimes the flares were worse, and it took months to recover, but this time was different. I was forced to sit on the couch for months on end watching *The Golden Girls*, contemplating where everything went wrong. I couldn't walk around and could only sit, stuck with my thoughts.

Why had it come to this? As a working parent and a powerful woman, why had I felt I couldn't put myself first? Why had my body been left in shambles? I was an independent person willing to work; why was I now not able to?

In our society, we are left fighting against an ineffectual care system, one that is not designed with wellness and prevention in mind. Our symptoms are often dismissed and covered up with pharmaceutical medications instead of searching for root causes. Insufficient funding is being provided for growing issues such as Lyme disease, MCAS, mold illness, and long COVID, and the rate of disability in this country is growing.

Our world—our environment and food—is becoming more toxic. Instead of arguing with each other, we should be spending more time and energy tracking down the harmful chemicals that are being inserted into our food supply. We should be funding extensive studies that examine the health of our soils and educating the world on disease prevention.

Instead, we live in a culture that places value on running yourself ragged, working late while only attaining four hours of sleep, and material items rather than true joy. Joy, what we need and want, is not obtained through material objects. It's a huge part of individual wellness for all. There needs to be a revolution wherein we as a society realize that we are cogs in an enormous machine and that the products of our manufacturing are materialistic. What feeds the soul, mind, and body?

My mind, body, and soul demanded a change. I couldn't push through anymore. Months turned into one year, then one year approached two years, and I was still not recovered. I required change—a life where I focused on the beauty around me and within myself. One where I would stop and get to know myself again, what I liked, and what brought me joy and inner peace. One where I could put myself and my health first.

Health is not just your physical well-being. It is all-encompassing. Health is your emotional health, spiritual health, financial health, environmental health, social health, intellectual health, and physical health. My body demanded that I explore each of those aspects and work toward living a more fulfilling life. I could no longer live on the fast-paced stressful highways with the majority. My body was suffering from inflammation, autoimmune disorders, and other complicated ailments that identified me as disabled. At first, the label was hard to swallow. It was especially tough to see it in writing once I was approved.

How can a successful mother with two young children suddenly stop in her tracks, slow down, and live a completely different life? I was conditioned to believe that life is supposed to be lived in the fast lane, always plugged in and connected, always hustling and making money and climbing the ladder. That's how we're supposed to live, right?

However, slowly, I began to appreciate that the universe had finally recognized my years and years of struggle to keep up with such a life. An approval of disability meant recognition that it was only becoming more difficult as the years went on to maintain such a lifestyle within a weakened body. If it meant I must be labeled as disabled for that to be acknowledged, then so be it. If that is what it took for me to make drastic life changes, then so be it. It was my only option left within the broken system.

I heard my body loud and clear and it was time to do just that. I left my job of sixteen years and began focusing exclusively on my health and wellness. I was determined to heal my body in every way possible.

For the first time in a long time, I was unsure of what lay ahead. I had no idea where life would take me, but I was excited to find out. Perhaps there would even be fewer storms to weather, and I could embrace the sun more often. It was time to live my life for me.

57

You Can Do This

IN JULY 2022, OUR FAMILY contracted COVID for the first time. We had done well up to that point, avoiding it due to my health conditions, but it finally caught up to us. It ripped through our household quickly, first infecting my weak immune system. Next, it infected John, and then Katie, and finally Marie.

Tremendous guilt washed over me as I knew I was the one who had caused it. I could have done better to protect myself and my household. I blamed my weak immune system for soaking up the virus and spreading it to everyone.

The next few weeks were torture. The kids were miserable with high fevers and vomiting and I could barely move. Thankfully, I was able to get Paxlovid for both me and John. I loaded the girls up with vitamins and supplements and hoped for the best. I resumed my spot on the couch, drinking liquids and using my nebulizer several times a day. It felt like I had been hit by a truck, knocking my recovery backward instead of propelling it forward. It became more and more difficult to breathe, and the chest congestion grew more pronounced each day. Luckily, the nebulizer was able to loosen up the mucus in my lungs, allowing me to cough and provide relief for my airway. As the weeks passed, we improved and eventually returned to normal.

One thing seemed to linger, however—John's fatigue. After dinner each night, John would find a spot on the couch and watch one of his favorite programs. Drained from his day at work, it was all he could do. His eyelids grew heavy, and his head would slowly fall forward as the fatigue took over. After letting him sleep for a while, I would wake him up to see if he wanted to go upstairs to bed. If not, he would stay on the couch.

I recovered from COVID well after a few months. All my issues that existed prior remained, but there were no lingering symptoms from the infection. I knew this had to be from the current protocol I was on due to my preexisting conditions. Every day I ate a clean mast cell diet, took h1 and h2 blockers, mast cell stabilizers, a multi-vitamin, hydroxychloroquine, and more. I'm sure this is what made my recovery different. I was already taking care of my body in the best way possible and focused heavily on recovery and wellness.

Still suffering from my existing health issues, I realized I was lucky I fared well with COVID. It could have been so much worse. I wondered: *Would I be so lucky next time? Why can't I get better? Am I permanently disabled? Is there a way to heal from this?* At each doctor's visit, the same words were repeated regarding MCAS, "This is a permanent condition for which there is no cure. All we can do is make you comfortable with medications." I didn't want to accept that. My situation was complex, but there was research being done every day. Doctors were educating themselves, conducting studies, and fighting the good fight for their patients. I was going to do the same for myself. It was time to buckle down and educate myself even further. My brain fog had shown some improvement, and I told myself: *You can do this. Let's learn all we can. It's time to find a doctor with the trifecta—an education on Lyme disease, MCAS, and mold illness. This is what needs to be done.*

So, I searched, and I searched. I read every article I could on MCAS, Lyme, and mold illness. I studied the connections, the root causes, and the complexities of the combination of these conditions. I watched videos, signed up for newsletters, read books, talked with patients of well-known specialists and read their medical evaluations, watched presentations by the top doctors in the field, and joined DrTalks.

By chance, DrTalks created a summit on the topic of MCAS, and it was scheduled for that month. I signed up immediately. Watching the summit provided me with the opportunity to listen to doctors from all over the country and beyond discuss the intricacies of MCAS, Lyme disease, mold illness, root causes, treatments, and the emotional trauma associated with all of it. It contained a wealth of new information and the names of additional medical professionals treating my conditions.

I continued my research, studying videos, opinions, and treatment methods of the doctors who were actively treating patients with all three conditions. I decided it was time to travel. I would find the doctor whose treatment methods and experiences spoke to me the most, and I would pay the money to travel for an appointment. There was nothing more my local doctors could do for me. They were out of ideas, and I had hit a wall with my treatment. This was the next step for me.

I chose three doctors that I liked and called their offices to discuss my case. For some of them, I would have to fly. For others, I would be able to pack up the camper and travel safely with all the accommodations to ensure my comfort. I settled on a doctor within an eight-hour drive from our town in Virginia. I had a strong connection with this doctor, and he had experience with all my issues. The visit would be expensive with a hefty first-time appointment fee, but I was willing to take the chance on him.

John and I packed up the camper in preparation for the trip, loading up my medications, dietary needs such as frozen chicken from the butcher, air purifier, and walker. We dropped the kids off at my mother's house, and we were off. I hadn't traveled a distance like this while dealing with all my new symptoms, and I knew I wouldn't fare well. One-hour trips to the doctor were enough to completely wipe me out and increase my neuropathy for weeks. This would be extremely tough on me, but it was to be one visit; subsequent visits would be done virtually. All I had to do was get through this one trip. I told myself again: *You can do this.*

The stress alone was enough to stir up my mast cells and cause an increase in symptoms. My body was completely unable to handle much stimulation, stress, or activity. With just a small amount, I'd be rendered useless and incapacitated. I hoped I'd made the right decision to travel so far and to pay so much money. I also hoped that the repercussions of my travels would be tolerable.

The trip turned out to be completely worth it! I conducted a new Igenex test on the spot, which I hadn't done in years. I was immediately placed on binders and tested again for mold exposure. This time, a more thorough and accurate testing method was used. I was asked to close my eyes and attempt to take a step. I immediately almost fell flat on my face. This was the first doctor to evaluate my balance and challenge my senses and abilities in a new way; the damage was evident. The lengthy visit felt worth every penny.

After the visit, John and I enjoyed a quiet night alone in the campground by the campfire. We tried to unwind from the day and prepare for the trip ahead. We had traveled eight hours just the day before, and we were about to do it again.

Recovering from our trip took about a month. It had been just as hard on me as I had expected. Three weeks after we returned home, I received my test results. The Igenex test revealed past infections of Lyme disease and babesia, which I already knew. However, it didn't reveal an active infection, which was good!

The mold test came back positive for several types of mycotoxins. "The term toxic mold is a bit misleading as it suggests that certain types of mold themselves are toxic. In reality, a very narrow set of molds produces secondary metabolites that produce toxins. These are known as mycotoxins. Studies show that more than fifty [percent] of homes and more than eighty-five [percent] of commercial buildings in the U.S. have water damage and mold. This is concerning since there is a strong likelihood that every [water-damaged] building also has the presence of mycotoxins."[34] I finally had confirmation of mold illness! It wasn't surprising considering all I had read. My prior LLMD had been correct when she had done that nasal swab a few years prior. We just needed a better test!

Since I was already on binders, it turned out this doctor had immediately placed me on the correct treatment. I continued to see this doctor virtually, trying one treatment at a time, some of which I reacted to. One medication plummeted my blood pressure to dangerous levels and almost resulted in another ER visit. Those

---

34 Jennifer, "The Ultimate Guide to Mycotoxins and What Makes Mold Toxic," Mold Help for You, May 12, 2022, https://rb.gy/ktt2pm.

with Lyme disease, Mast Cell Activation Syndrome, and various other misunderstood chronic illnesses tend to avoid the ER at all costs and will hold out until it's absolutely necessary. Another medication caused extreme hypoglycemia within two hours of consumption. Trial and error can be scary and time-consuming for a patient with MCAS as we are sensitive to many triggers and substances, even in small amounts.

Since I was positive for mycotoxins, I pondered what sort of damage this had done to my immune system and which of my symptoms were caused by mold illness. I pictured the many leaks at my workplace and wondered how much mold was lurking beneath the cubicle walls, carpet, and ceiling tiles.

Eager to learn more, I returned to the DrTalks MCAS Summit and re-watched the videos on mold. All of them. I researched, read books and articles, and sought out the knowledge of ISEAI (International Society for Environmentally Acquired Illness) professionals.

It became quite evident that mold is a complex issue that is difficult for the average person to navigate. As mold is a relatively common occurrence in homes and commercial buildings, I was perplexed to learn that there are no EPA regulations or standards. Of course, this leads to an unregulated industry, a lack of accountability, and a plethora of mold professionals with improper training. Simply put, they don't know what they don't know.

Individuals experiencing mold contamination within their homes or workplaces are sometimes left with subpar mold professionals and inadequate, unsatisfactory remediation.

If you dive into this realm, be prepared to be met with predatory behavior and sales tactics that will leave you appalled.

Despite homes being considered "clear" of mold following remediation, many sensitive homeowners remain sick and are left wondering why. This can be the result of inadequate testing, a failed visual inspection, the lack of a small particle cleaning, or just a complex mold issue that's difficult to uncover, to name a few.[35] A

---

[35] Inadequate testing can be described as utilizing solely ambient (collected from the middle of the room) air samples with no additional air samples, swabs, or tape testing. Also, conducting no further investigation behind walls and ceilings when appropriate can

small particle cleaning ensures the removal of any dead or dormant mold that has not yet sporulated.

Should inactive mold become wet, it can sporulate and turn active. Mold can actually survive on surfaces that are not visibly wet, as it extracts moisture from the air. All it takes is high humidity for mold to grow and flourish. This is why it's recommended to maintain a humidity of thirty to fifty percent within your home.

Furthermore, inactive mold can get into the air and cause health issues for humans, particularly for sensitive individuals. In fact, mold in this state is lighter and becomes airborne more easily, seeking out favorable conditions for its survival. Mold colonies can even communicate with each other through chemical signals! They reproduce through tiny spores that can become airborne, facilitating their spread.

When we heat our homes in the winter, hot air rises, escaping or leaking through the unsealed parts of our home in the attic above. When air leaves a home, new air replaces it by coming in through cracks and holes toward the lower part of the home. This process is referred to as the stack effect. As a result of this repeated process, mold spores rise to other levels of your home along with the warm currents. Consequently, air quality in your basement or crawlspace is important as it affects the indoor air quality and health of the rest of your home.

Fifty percent of the air we breathe throughout the day comes from the basement or crawlspace. In the summer, the opposite occurs with cool air leaking through the bottom and entering at the top. How air moves through your home and the condition of your HVAC system and its air ducts plays a huge role in the health of your home and the distribution of mold spores. Improper cleaning of air ducts during remediation, for example, will also contribute to the mold issue. If the remediation process is done incorrectly, mold spores will continue to spread by way of the stack effect and through your HVAC system, exacerbating the problem. Homes and

---

result in undiscovered hidden mold. Testing can include wall cavity testing or John Banta's pathway testing. Air moves through your walls, exiting electrical outlets to mix with your breathable air. Think of your home as a living breathing ecosystem, or your own personal habitat.

commercial buildings are often improperly cleared, requiring additional more thorough remediation.

John continued to go to work, despite his fatigue. He brushed it off and assumed it would take him longer to recover from COVID than the rest of us. He was now running his own mechanic business and was the sole owner and employee. Taking time off was not an option. It was then I noticed a change in Marie, and my focus completely shifted from John's fatigue to Marie's symptoms. She had become more irritable and tired and had developed extreme acne on her face and shoulders. On occasion, she would throw up or complain of stomach pain after eating. The subtle changes and symptoms may have been easily dismissed by someone else, but I knew something wasn't right. I could feel it in my gut.

I scheduled yearly physicals for both Katie and Marie and headed to their primary care physician. During the appointment, I expressed concern regarding the changes I had seen in Marie. Why was her acne so bad? Could this be food allergies? I was quickly dismissed, and she was prescribed cream for the acne. Convinced it was just puberty, they sent us on our way with the prescription and nothing else.

It was what happened next that terrified me.

Marie awoke from sleep one morning and stumbled downstairs rubbing her eyes. Walking into the kitchen where I was making breakfast, Marie mumbled, "Mom, my face feels swollen. Can you look at it?"

"Sure, honey, let me take a look."

As Marie came closer, my eyes grew wide with fear.

"Mom! Why are you looking at me like that? You're scaring me."

I couldn't hide my fear and worry. I was never good at concealing my emotions. I quickly attempted to change my facial expression and examined Marie.

"Well, your face is swollen, honey. Come closer, let me see. Did you eat something different last night?"

"No. I don't know."

"Are you having any trouble breathing or swallowing?"

"No. Why would I?" Marie took off running toward the downstairs bathroom and looked at herself in the mirror.

I followed her and stood in the doorway. Tears welled up in Marie's eyes as she stared at her reflection.

"Why does my face look like this?"

"I'm not sure. Are you feeling anything else right now?" My fear was anaphylaxis. I had suffered from anaphylaxis in the past, but my face had never grown as swollen as hers. Her lips were puffed and one eye was nearly shut. I took comfort in knowing I had an EpiPen close by. Since we nearly matched in weight now, the adult dose should be okay. I realized I didn't have the answer to that for sure, so I hoped she wouldn't need it.

"I'm so itchy, and I have these," Marie said as she lifted her leg and presented it to me.

As I examined her, I noticed hives. They were everywhere. I began to examine her entire body and saw hives on her arms, neck, back, and stomach.

"Everything is going to be okay, honey. Let's get you some medicine to take away that itching."

Trying not to panic, I went through the cabinets, searching for the children's Benadryl. We were out. How could that be? I always kept medicine on hand. After continuing to push aside other medications, I finally came across Zyrtec. It would have to do for now.

"Here, take this. It will help."

Marie relaxed on the couch as I made phone calls to doctors and tried to get her an appointment.

As luck would have it, the local allergist's office had a cancellation and was able to get Marie in for a new patient appointment!

Thrilled, we rushed there the next day.

As Marie sat on the examination table filled with anxiety, the doctor examined the hives on her arms and legs.

"Hmmm. I'm not quite sure what this is. Does she have a virus?"

"No. None of us are sick right now. We homeschool and haven't seen anyone else in days. Could it be food allergies or some sort of flea or insect bites?"

"No, I doubt that. She must have a virus. I would continue with the Zyrtec and add Claritin. Give her Claritin in the morning, and Zyrtec before bed. You can go ahead and give her Benadryl also as needed."

"It's safe to take that many antihistamines?"

"Yeah, it won't hurt her."

"But what about food allergies? Could they cause a rash like this?"

"I doubt it. We could test her for food allergies, but not right now since she's on antihistamines. They must be out of her system for several days before testing. We could do a blood test for wheat, but I don't think it's necessary."

That was the dumbest thing I ever heard. Why wouldn't you be able to test for food allergies while on antihistamines? What if you need antihistamines to prevent anaphylaxis? Did they not see how swollen her face was?

"How did you all get an appointment today? I haven't seen you before. You must be new patients."

Perplexed by her question, I answered, "Your office had a cancellation today."

"Interesting," she replied with a raised eyebrow.

The nurse and doctor abruptly ended the conversation and ushered us toward the door.

"It was good to see you today. Keep taking those antihistamines and call us if you have any questions."

Once again, my concerns about food allergies were brushed aside, and we were sent home with the suggestion of medication and no answers. We were ushered in, placed on an assembly line for our fifteen-minute appointment, and then sent packing.

Marie and I made our way out to the car and sat in the parking lot. I stared out the window in disbelief. I reached over my shoulder and pulled down the seatbelt. As I buckled, my thoughts clicked together too. I realized the system was repeating itself—with my daughter.

"Let's go, Mom. I'm ready to get out of here."

"Okay, let's go."

I would not let this happen to her too. The next day, I would insist that her primary care doctor test her for food allergies.

I sent a few messages back and forth on the patient portal and was eventually successful. We tested her for food allergies, and the results were in.

She had every single major food allergy. All of them. Peanuts, soy, wheat, milk, eggs, fish—How could this be? What child suddenly develops this level of food allergies out of nowhere?

That's when I knew. I knew the answer.

It was my greatest fear.

It was Lyme disease.

It was time to test her again. These were the signs. I couldn't ignore them. No mainstream medical doctor was going to understand. It was time to bring in the doctors I trusted most. After making a few calls, I was able to find a doctor to do a blood draw for Igenex. As I awaited the results, I feared the worst. If this test came back positive, I didn't think I could handle it. This would be what finally destroyed me. What if COVID had reactivated congenital Lyme? We had been lucky all these years that she lived a healthy life, free of symptoms, or so I thought.

I replayed her entire life in my mind. The positive cord blood testing, the exam for Lyme disease as an infant, her change in temperament around age five, how she struggled to learn and stay focused in school, and how she seemed to react to certain foods, sometimes with vomiting. Strawberries and cheese had been potential suspects in the past, but the reactions were too infrequent to have me convinced. What if the subtle signs had been there all along, and I had missed them? There was no missing them now. I feared Lyme disease was staring me in the face. My greatest enemy and my greatest fear, infecting my greatest love, my child.

As we awaited the test results, Marie's symptoms increased. One morning she came downstairs and told me she was feeling faint. Instantly, her face turned pale and her lips slightly blue. I knew what was coming.

"We need to lay you down, Marie, right now."

I managed to get her flat, reassuring her and calmly waiting to see if syncope was inevitable. I'd hoped my quick action would prevent it as I knew from experience syncope at a young age can be traumatizing. Once the feeling started to pass, she sipped some water. I had her eat a snack and remain on the sofa a while longer. She started to feel better.

In the days following the pre-syncopal episode, Marie struggled with extreme fatigue, increased hives, swelling of her ankles and face, bouts of crying and profound sadness, outbursts of anger, and weakness in her legs. We had removed gluten from her diet, but I knew we wouldn't see results overnight. Slowly, we were subtracting other food items from her diet. Going gluten-free alone is difficult for an adult, let alone a child.

Despite all that we were experiencing, we attempted camping trips and occasional outings as a family. We were determined to continue to live our lives, just at a slower pace than a healthy family would—and with a lot more pills in tow! Marie often complained about weakness in her legs and would announce, "My legs are done. Can we go home?" It broke my heart to hear that as I knew it all too well. Using a cane or a walker, I wondered if I should get her the same. Instead, we would immediately stop and rest until her legs felt a little better. I wanted the girls to have time to be a kid and days not to be filled with only symptoms and medication.

Our trips looked a little different with frequent rest required and only one activity a day at most. That was okay. We were able to enjoy a change in scenery, time by the ocean, campground fires, lakes, mountains, and small adventures. These were our adventures, no matter how small. Positive family memories among the chaos gave us something to look forward to.

A few weeks later, the test results were in. I locked myself in my bedroom for privacy. This was it.

I clicked on the test, and it opened.

Lyme ImmunoBlot IgM
IGX Criteria: **Positive**
CDC/NYS Criteria: **Positive**

Lyme ImmunoBlot IgG
IGX Criteria: Negative
CDC/NYS Criteria: Negative

Babesia ImmunoBlot IgM: Negative
Babesia ImmunoBlot IgG: Negative
Bartonella ImmunoBlot IgM: Negative
*Bartonella ImmunoBlot IgG: **Positive***

My heart sank.

A positive, active Lyme infection and Bartonella.

I collapsed to my knees.

My chest heaved in and out as I sobbed on my bedroom floor. The world spun around me and collapsed on top of my broken soul. Just as I had predicted, I did not take it well.

For days, I cried. I cried, and I cried, and I sobbed, and I wept. I knew a difficult road stretched ahead for us. *How were we going to get through this? What doctor should she see? How were we going to afford this?* My heart broke and shattered into a tiny million pieces. Soul-crushing guilt consumed me. I had done this. It was congenital Lyme, wasn't it? Long COVID was bringing it to the surface. I had tested every tick she had ever had on her, and they had all been negative. This was my fault.

Why had John picked me? Why had we married? Why had he had kids with me? He had picked the wrong woman. This was all on me. Everything was on me. These were my thoughts as my guilt slowly crushed me, squeezing out any bit of strength I had left.

Days went by. Unable to function, I wallowed in my culpability and pain. Slowly, I realized, the only way out was through. This was another storm. I had to hunker down again.

I brushed myself off and stood up.

"You can do this, Kristin! Get up! Move forward! It's time to help your daughter. You're the only one who can," I said out loud to myself.

And so, one foot in front of the other, I did.

RESOURCES

Below is a list of resources for the curious. It is in no way a personal endorsement. Doing your due diligence, checking qualifications, and following your gut is critical. These websites are great starting points for those seeking answers.

You must take everything with a grain of salt and cross-check data and information. Listen to your gut. Remain alert and always keep in mind that some may try to take advantage of your situation.

As always, discuss any medical issues with a medical professional you can trust.

Lyme Disease

Bay Area Lyme Foundation
Bayarealyme.org

Bill Rawls Treatment Guide
Rawlsmd.com/treatment-guide

BioMed Publishing Group
Lymebook.com

The California Lyme Disease Association
Lymedisease.org

Center for Lyme Action
Centerforlymeaction.org

Columbia University – Lyme and Tick-borne Disease Research Center
Columbia-lyme.org

DNA Connexions (Lyme Urine Test)
Dnaconnexions.com

Joseph Burrascano Symptom Checklist
lymedisease.org/wp-
content/uploads/2015/02/Symptomchecklist-burrascano.pdf

IGeneX Inc.
Igenex.com

International Lyme and Associated Diseases Society
ILADS.org

LivLyme Foundation
Livlymefoundation.org
Grants for patients 21 and under

LymeAid 4 Kids
lymediseaseassociation.org/grants/lymeaid-4-kids/about-lyme-
aid-4-kids/
Grants $1,000 for patients 21 and under without insurance

Lyme Basics
Lymebasics.org
Formerly known as the Lyme Disease Association of Southeastern
Pennsylvania (LDASEPA)

Lyme Disease Association
Lymediseaseassociation.org

Lyme Disease Network
Lymenet.org

Lyme Info
Lymeinfo.net

Lyme Light Foundation
Lymelightfoundation.org
Grants for patients 25 and under

Lyme Treatment Foundation
Lymetreatementfoundation.org
Grants for patient costs associated with an LLMD

Medical Diagnostic Laboratory
Mdlab.com

NatCapLyme
Natcaplyme.org

Project Lyme
Projectlyme.org

Stony Brook University
Renaissance.stonybrookmedicine.edu/pathology/tick

Vibrant Wellness
Vibrant-wellness.com

POTS/Dysautonomia

Dysautonomia Information Network
Dinet.org

Dysautonomia International
Dysautonomiainternational.org

Dysautonomia Support Network
Dysautonomiasupport.org

POTs Treatment Center
Potstreatmentcenter.com

Standing up to POTs
Standinguptopots.org

Low-Histamine Food Lists

Bev's SIGHI Food List
Rider4health.org

The Histamine & Tyramine Restricted Diet
Jillcarnahna.com

Intolerances App
iOS or Google Play store (blue with a strawberry symbol)

Mast Cell 360
Mastcell360.com

MCAS

Aim Center – Dr. Lawrence Afrin
Aimcenterpm.com

Dr. Becky Campbell
Drbeckycampbell.com

Beth O'Hara, FN
Mastcell360.com

Christine Schaffner, ND
Drchristineschaffner.com

Global Classification of Mast Cell Activation Disorders: An ICD-10-CM-Adjusted Proposal of the ECNM-AIM Consortium
https://rb.gy/rq7r82

How Mast Cell Activation Syndrome, Mitochondrial Dysfunction, and the Brain Impact Your Patients
https://rb.gy/7eb38k

The Mast Cell Disease Society
Tmsforacure.org

Mast Cells: Normal Role, Allergies, Anaphylaxis, MCAS & Mastocytosis
https://rb.gy/krvwkb

Robert Miller, CTN
Tolhealth.com

Dr. Tania Dempsey
Drtaniadempsey.com

Wine Wand
Wine Purifier & Sulfite Remover
Drinkpurewine.com

Documentaries

I'm Not Crazy, I'm Sick
Available on Amazon Prime

MCAS/EDS/POTS Documentary
Ldnresearchtrust.org/documentary-fundraiser

The Monster Inside Me
Themonsterinsideme.com

The Quiet Epidemic
Available on Amazon Prime

Under Our Skin
Available on Amazon Prime

Meat Frozen After Slaughter

North Star Bison
Northstarbison.com

White Oak Pastures
Whiteoakpastures.com

Wild Fork
Wildforkfoods.com

Mold/Mycotoxins

American Council for Accredited Certification
ACAC.org

Andrew Campbell
Andrewcampbellmd.com

Benefect Decon 30
Benefect.com

BioZaq Poly (Water-Soluble Laundry Bags)
Biozaq.com

Black Diamond Services
Blackdiamondservices.com

Canine Mold Detective
Caninemolddetective.com

EnviroBiomics, Inc.
Envirobiomics.com

Healing from Mold
Healingfrommold.org

Home Cleanse
Homecleanse.com

ImmunoLytics
Immunolytics.com

International Society for Environmentally Acquired Illness
Iseai.org

Mast Cell 360
Mastcell360.com

May Dooley: Mold Control on a Budget
Moldcontrolonabudget.com

Micro Balance
Microbalancehealthproducts.com

Mold Canine
Moldcanine.com

Mold Dog
Mold-dog.com

Mold Dog Knows
Molddogknows.com

Montana Basement Solutions
Montanabasementsolutions.com

My Chemical-Free House
Mychemicalfreehouse.net/2019/01/the-best-air-purifiers-for-mould-review.html

Mycometrics
Mycometrics.com

MyMycoLab
Mymycolab.com

Neil Nathan Trained Practitioners
Neilnathanmd.com/books/

RealTime Laboratories
Realtimelab.com

RespirareLabs
Respirarelabs.com

Surviving Mold
Survivingmold.com/resources-for-patients/treatment

Surviving Toxic Mold
Survivingtoxicmold.com/saving_your_possessions

Toxic Mould Support Australia
Toxicmould.org/mould-101-preventing-removing-and-remediating

We Inspect
Yesweinspect.com

WelEssence
Riehydroxyls.com

Books

Accessing the Healing Power of the Vagus Nerve
Stanley Rosenberg

Bitten
Kris Newby

Chronic
Steven Phillips and Dana Parish

Coping with Lyme Disease: A Practical Guide to Dealing with Diagnosis and Treatment
Denise Lang with Kenneth Leigner

Cure Unknown
Pam Weintraub

Dirty Genes
Ben Lynch

Healing Lyme: Natural Healing of Lyme Borreliosis and the Coinfections Chlamydia and Spotted Fever Rickettsiosis
Stephen Buhner

The Healthy House: How to Buy One, How to Build One, How to Cure a Sick One
John Bower

How Can I Get Better? An Action Plan for Treating Resistant Lyme & Chronic Disease
Richard Horowitz

Lyme Brain
Nicola McFadzean Ducharme

Never Bet Against Occam
Lawrence B. Afrin

Prescriptions for a Healthy House: A Practical Guide for Architects, Builders, and Homeowners
Paula Baker-Laporte and John Banta

The Top 10 Lyme Disease Treatments: Defeat Lyme Disease with the Best of Conventional and Alternative Medicine
Bryan Rosner

Toxic: Heal Your Body from Mold Toxicity, Lyme Disease, Multiple Chemical Sensitivities and Chronic Environmental Illness
Neil Nathan

UnLocking Lyme: Myths, Truths, and Practical Solutions for Chronic Lyme Disease
William Rawls

When Antibiotics Fail: Lyme Disease and Rife Machines with Critical Evaluation of Leading Alternative Therapies
Bryan Rosner

Why Can't I Get Better? Solving the Mystery of Lyme and Chronic Disease
Richard Horowitz

Tick Testing

Connecticut Veterinary Medical Diagnostic Laboratory
Cvmdl.uconn.edu

ECO Laboratory
Ticktests.com

Igenex
Igenez.com/tick-test/

Pennsylvania Tick Research Lab
Ticklab.org

TickCheck: Pennsylvania Tick Testing Laboratory
Tickcheck.com

Ticknology
Ticknology.org

TickReport
Tickreport.com

Limbic System Retraining

Annie Hopper: Dynamic Neural Retraining System (DNRS)
Retrainingthebrain.com

Re-origin
Re-origin.com

Safe & Sounds Protocol (SSP): Unyte
Integratedlistening.com

The Gupta Program
Guptaprogram.com

Electrical Muscle Stimulation

E Stim and Movement Essentials E Course
Terrywahls.com/estimcourse

ABOUT THE AUTHOR

Kristin Parthemos is a wife and mother of two young girls. She holds a Bachelor's degree in Legal Studies from the University of Maryland Global Campus, a Paralegal Certificate, and is a Certified Integrative Nutrition Health Coach. She began her career as a paralegal at a private law firm and then worked for the FBI for sixteen years. She then followed her passion for helping others achieve health and wellness and currently owns her own Health Coaching business, Health & Harmony LLC.

When not working, you'll find her homeschooling her two children. In her spare time, she enjoys creating meals in the kitchen, camping with her family, writing, painting, meditating, and enjoying time in nature.

To connect with Kristin, visit her at healthandharmonyhc.com.

www.ingramcontent.com/pod-product-compliance
Lightning Source LLC
Chambersburg PA
CBHW020445130626
46549CB00001B/310